LABORATORY ANIMALS IN VACCINE PRODUCTION AND CONTROL

DEVELOPMENTS IN HEMATOLOGY AND IMMUNOLOGY

Lijnen, H.R., Collen, D. and Verstraete, M., eds: Synthetic Substrates in Clinical Blood Coagulation Assays. 1980. ISBN 90-247-2409-0

Smit Sibinga, C.Th., Das, P.C. and Forfar, J.O., eds: Paediatrics and Blood Transfusion. 1982. ISBN 90-247-2619-0

Fabris, N., ed: Immunology and Ageing. 1982. ISBN 90-247-2640-9

Hornstra, G.: Dietary Fats, Prostanoids and Arterial Thrombosis. 1982. ISBN 90-247-2667-0

Smit Sibinga, C.Th., Das, P.C. and Loghem, van J.J., eds: Blood Transfusion and Problems of Bleeding. 1982. ISBN 90-247-3058-9

Dormandy, J., ed: Red Cell Deformability and Filterability. 1983. ISBN 0-89838-578-4

Smit Sibinga, C.Th., Das, P.C. and Taswell, H.F., eds: Quality Assurance in Blood Banking and Its Clinical Impact. 1984. ISBN 0-89838-618-7

Besselaar, A.M.H.P. van den, Gralnick, H.R. and Lewis, S.M., eds: Thromboplastin Calibration and Oral Anticoagulant Control. 1984. ISBN 0-89838-637-3

Fondu, P. and Thijs, O., eds: Haemostatic Failure in Liver Disease. 1984. ISBN 0-89838-640-3

Smit Sibinga, C.Th., Das, P.C. and Opelz, G., eds: Transplantation and Blood Transfusion. 1984. ISBN 0-89838-686-1

Schmid-Schönbein, H., Wurzinger, L.J. and Zimmerman, R.E., eds: Enzyme Activation in Blood-Perfused Artificial Organs. 1985. ISBN 0-89838-704-3

Dormandy, J., ed: Blood Filtration and Blood Cell Deformability. 1985. ISBN 0-89838-714-0

Smit Sibinga, C.Th., Das, P.C. and Seidl, S., eds: Plasma Fractionation and Blood Transfusion. 1985. ISBN 0-89838-761-2

Dawids, S. and Bantjes, A., eds: Blood Compatible Materials and their Testing. 1986. ISBN 0-89838-813-9

Smit Sibinga, C.Th., Das, P.C. and Greenwalt, T.J., eds: Future Developments in Blood Banking. 1986. ISBN 0-89838-824-4

Berlin, A., Dean, J., Draper, M.H., Smith, E.M.B. and Spreafico, F., eds: Immunotoxicology. 1987. ISBN 0-89838-843-0

Ottenhoff, T. and De Vries, R.: Recognition of *M. leprae* antigens. 1987. ISBN 0-89838-887-2

Touraine, J.-L., Gale, R.P. and Kochupillai, V., eds: Fetal Liver Transplantation. 1987. ISBN 0-89838-975-5

Smit Sibinga, C.Th., Das, P.C. and Engelfriet, C.P., eds: White cells and platelets in blood transfusion. 1987. ISBN 0-89838-976-3

Hendriksen, C.F.M.: Laboratory animals in vaccine production and control. 1988. ISBN 0-89838-398-6

Laboratory animals in vaccine production and control

Replacement, reduction and refinement

by

COENRAAD F.M. HENDRIKSEN

National Institute of Public Health and Environmental Protection,
The Netherlands

Preface by

JOHN C. PETRICCIANI

Chief Biologicals,
World Health Organization

KLUWER ACADEMIC PUBLISHERS
DORDRECHT / BOSTON / LONDON

Library of Congress Cataloging in Publication Data

```
Hendriksen, Coenraad F. M.,
    Laboratory animals in vaccine production and control :
  replacement, reduction, and refinement / Coenraad F.M. Hendriksen.
        p.   cm. -- (Developments in hematology and immunology)
    Includes bibliographies.

    1. Vaccines--Synthesis.  2. Vaccines--Testing.  3. Animal
  experimentation.   I. Title.  II. Series.
  QR189.H47 1988
  615'.372--dc19                                          88-19721
                                                              CIP
```

ISBN-13: 978-94-010-7088-1   e-ISBN-13: 978-94-009-1321-9

DOI: 10.1007/978-94-009-1321-9

Published by Kluwer Academic Publishers,
P.O. Box 17, 3300 AA Dordrecht, The Netherlands.

Kluwer Academic Publishers incorporates
the publishing programmes of
D. Reidel, Martinus Nijhoff, Dr W. Junk and MTP Press.

Sold and distributed in the U.S.A. and Canada
by Kluwer Academic Publishers,
101 Philip Drive, Norwell, MA 02061, U.S.A.

In all other countries, sold and distributed
by Kluwer Academic Publishers Group,
P.O. Box 322, 3300 AH Dordrecht, The Netherlands.

Translation: Hetty Volman, Bilthoven

"PUT THE BLUE
OF THE SEA
AGAINST THE
BLUE OF
THE SKY,
ADD SOME WHITE
FOR A SAIL,
AND SOON THE
WIND WILL RISE"

(W. Hussem, 1965)

To Nina, who else

ACKNOWLEDGEMENTS

Research for this book was undertaken in the National Institute of Public Health and Environmental Protection (RIVM), the Netherlands, and several other institutes.
I owe a debt to all those individuals who helped me with their stimulating contributions and constructive criticism. Contact with the following persons has been of particular importance:
- Dr.J.G.Kreeftenberg, Head of the Laboratory for Control of Bacterial Vaccines, National Institute of Public Health and Environmental Protection (RIVM), the Netherlands;
- Dr.W.J.Pereboom, Laboratory Animal Department, Duphar B.V., the Netherlands;
- Prof.Dr.H.Rozemond, Veterinary Public Health Inspectorate, Animal Experimentation Department, the Netherlands;
- Prof.Dr.L.F.M.van Zutphen, Department Laboratory Animal Studies, State University of Utrecht, the Netherlands.

Much of the manuscript was typed by Mrs.H.A.J.P.Averson-Hulshof and Mrs.V.L.H.Wauben and my thanks are due to them for their excellent work, cheerfulness and reliability.

CONTENTS

PREFACE

In recent years there has been a great deal of international
public debate, unrest, and perhaps more than anything else,
misunderstanding regarding the use of animals in research and
testing. Within the animal rights movement, the debate and
disagreement tend to focus on what appear to be three mutually
exclusive approaches: 1) regulate the use of animals through
legislation; 2) abolish the use of animals altogether; and 3)
search for alternatives to the use of animals. While it may be
convenient to think in terms of unique solutions to problems, and
while each of the above approaches has a special appeal to
certain individuals, it is not very helpful to animals, science,
or the public to suggest that any of those options is the only
way to proceed. Complex problems rarely have simple answers, and
this is as true in the case of animals in research and testing as
it is for other issues.
In order to replace animals in various tests, there must be an
effort aimed at finding valid alternatives to the use of animals.
To suggest that all the alternatives already exist is either
terribly naive or terribly misleading. What is true is that a
variety of techniques are available which might be applied to
specific tests in which animals are now used. But to validate
those alternatives takes time, personnel and money. It is also
important to note that because technology keeps evolving at such
a rapid rate, what seems impractical if not impossible today, may
become possible next month or next year. This in turn means we
must constantly reassess which animal tests are candidates for
replacement.
The large majority of society wants products which have been
tested for safety and effectiveness. At the same time, animal
rights groups want to eliminate all painful testing. By working
together, ways can be explored to reconcile these apparently
conflicting aims. It takes a willingness to understand differing
points of view. It takes an effort to see that there are common
interests and that common ground for working out solutions does
exist. And it takes patience along with compromise.
This book presents a unique collection of information which is
relevant to all those who are concerned with vaccine production,
control, and use. It is unique in both its content as well as in
the background which led to its publication because it represents
an example of how government and animal rights groups have worked
together succesfully on a scientifically sound project.
The World Health Organization has been interested for many years
in the possibilities of replacing the animal tests which are
specified in its international Requirements for vaccines with
alternate in vitro tests; and some progress has already been made
in that respect. This volume provides a substantial amount of
material for discussion among experts, and for further refinement
so as to ultimately result in additional internationally
acceptable tests which do not use animals or which reduce the
number of animals, but which also provide assurance that vaccines
are both safe and potent.

John C. Petricciani, M.D.   Summer 1987
Chief, Biologicals
World Health Organization

Laboratory animals are still used extensively in biomedical
research although a tendency towards reduction can be noted.
Animal experimentation is a frequent subject of discussion in
society, and there is a growing feeling that it is undesirable on
ethical grounds. In public circles, the argument understandably
centres on animal experiments that are morally and scientifically
questionable, such as the LD50 test or the Draize test. However,
generalization can distort the overall picture of animal research
because it also questions the use of animals for justified and
essential research. It cannot be denied that a large part of
modern health care is based on knowledge acquired through
experiments on live animals. It should also not be forgotten that
biomedical research is governed by social priorities. One example
is the social pressure for safe and effective products so that we
are faced with the parodox that the critics of animal research
are alsoe frequently, although unwittingly, the initiators of
this type of research.
Nevertheless, the growing public awakening to the permissibility
of animal studies and the way they are performed should be taken
seriously. If we regard (vertebrate) animals as suitable
substitutes for human beings in medical research because of their
close relationship to man, both physiologically and anatomically,
then the same reasoning should motivate us to use them prudently.
The scientific community too is aware that an experimental animal
is more than merely an instrument. This observation requires some
explanation. The animal experimenter is still all too often
regarded as the pre-eminent supporter of animal research. The
fact that many researchers are highly committed to their work
does not imply that they are therefore indifferent to the fate of
the experimental animal. Still, the author believes that, more
than has been the case thus far, this attitude should find
expression in practice and a balance should be sought between the
scientist's research and social responsibility, on the one hand,
and his moral responsibility towards the animal, on the other.
The law can give us some guidelines but it should be remembered
that it can do no more than that. The attention of the individual
scientist to the ethical aspects of his research on animals is of
vital importance, manifesting itself in, among other things, a
continual reviewing of his research in order to replace, reduce
and refine the use of experimental animals as much as possible.
This approach is of particular interest because this emphasizing
of ethical principles is accompanied by maintenance of the
scientific value of research, while it may at the same time also
lead to evident economic benefits.
Therefore, "alternative methods", that is, any procedures by
which a replacement, reduction and/or refinement have been
achieved in the use of experimental animals are an excellent
basis for science as well as for animal protection, industry and
government.
Alternatives can have special significance particularly in those
fields of biomedical research where the use of animals is
controlled by stringent national, international and supranational
laws and guidelines, such as for toxicity testing and vaccine
control. If new alternatives can find acceptance here, leading to
the replacement, reduction and refinement of the use of living
animals for research, their impact will be great.

1

2

On the premise that even regulated, routine animal experiments
are more than just a "routine" matter, a project was launched in
the Netherlands to study the opportunities for replacing,
reducing and refining animal experiments, also known as the three
Rs. The project was confined to vaccine production and quality
control, where many animals are used, often in a routine manner
as prescribed by legislation.
It should be stressed that the project is unique, not only for
the Netherlands but also in an international context, because it
embodied the cooperation of the authorities, industry and the
animal protection groups in the Netherlands.
The objective of the survey was to find an answer to the
following questions:
 - What is the importance of animals in the production and
   quality control of vaccines?
 - Which vaccines are involved?
 - How are the tests for vaccine control performed in various
   countries and in particular in the Netherlands?
 - Which studies are being undertaken to replace animals in
   vaccine control?
 - What procedures inflicting less distress are being
   investigated?
 - What national, international and supranational guidelines and
   regulations exist for tests on vaccines?
 - How are guidelines and regulations drawn up and how can they
   be adapted or changed?
This book represents the final report of the survey. As many
aspects as possible of the three Rs - replacement, reduction and
refinement - were examined as regards the development, production
and control of vaccines. Chapters 2 and 3 outline the historical
development of the use of animals for the purpose of the
production and quality control of vaccines. Chapters 4 and 5 deal
with current vaccine research and the importance of its various
methodologies involving laboratory animals, and chapters 6 and 7
describe the growing interest in "alternative" methods. A summary
of the existing national, international and supranational
guidelines for testing vaccines is given in chapters 8-12, while
the opportunities for replacing, reducing or refining the use of
experimental animals in the production and quality control of
bacterial and viral vaccines for human and veterinary use are
also considered in these chapters. Chapter 13 discusses possible
future developments in the production and control of vaccines.
Finally, chapter 14 summarizes the recommendations resulting from
this report.
Research on animals for the production and control of vaccines
has a history of a hundred years, to which thousands of
scientists have contributed. It will be obvious that one
literature study cannot solve the controversial issue of the
value of experimental animals for research. However, if the
suggestions made here are implemented, the use of laboratory
animals can be substantially reduced.

CHAPTER 2: ANIMAL EXPERIMENTATION AND THE DEVELOPMENT OF
VACCINES: A BRIEF HISTORICAL OUTLINE

According to the annual registration of the use of laboratory
animals in the Netherlands, 251,000 animals were used in this
country in 1986 for the production, testing and biological
standardization of biological products, including vaccines in
particular (1). The total figure for that year in the Netherlands
was about 1.21 millions.
The total number of laboratory animals used throughout the world
and for what purpose is not known. Rough estimates, based on
assumptions rather than on data, vary between 100 and 200
millions a year.
When seeking an answer to the hows and whys of such extensive
practice, one is inevitably referred to history. It is difficult
to explain the present without knowledge of the past, and this is
especially true of the use of laboratory animals which is so
closely linked to other developments.
The following brief historical account is intended to provide
some background information about the importance of the
experimental animal in the development and routine testing of
sera and vaccines.

1. THE ANCIENT WORLD

It is generally assumed that animal experiments were first
performed in ancient Greece. Mysticism and superstition in
medicine were here gradually replaced by a natural-philosophical
approach, where observation and experimentation became the
important elements. The very first animal experiments known to us
are the physiological investigations by Alkmaeon of Kroton (550-
500 B.C.) (2).

2. THE 19th CENTURY

2.1. Claude Bernard
However, it was not until the middle of the last century that
animal experimentation acquired a fully fledged scientific status
in biomedical research. This development can be largely
attributed to the Frenchman Claude Bernard. He came up against
the inconstancy of physiological phenomena, which he ascribed to
the large variety of factors affecting the course of an
experiment. He formulated the basic principles for a rational
approach to animal experimentation in his classic works entitled
"Introduction à l'étude de la médecine expérimentale" (3) and
"Principes de médecine expérimentale" (4).
His ideas on how to formulate scientific questions, standardize
an experimental design, choose an animal species, and ensure a
high reproducibility are still relevant. He was convinced that
animal experimentation was valuable to biomedical research. This
is what he said on this subject in 1865: "The results of animal
experiments are, from a physiological, pathological and
therapeutic point of view, not only important for fundamental
medical research, but I even believe that applied medical
research can never develop into a mature science without this
comparative research on animals" (3).
These comparative studies, initiated by Bernard, have undeniably
deepened our understanding of the origin, course and prevention

3

of infectious diseases. It contributed to refuting the theory of
spontaneous generation, that is, the concept that microorganisms
generate from non-living matter.

2.2. Louis Pasteur and Robert Koch

It was Louis Pasteur (1822-1895) and Robert Koch (1843-1910) who,
using Bernard's concepts on experimental animal research,
succeeded in underpinning scientifically and experimentally the
causal connection between infectious diseases and microorganisms.
Koch's postulates, stated lucidly in his 1884 study "The
aetiology of tuberculosis" (5), have been of fundamental
importance as regards the role of experimental animals in this.
These postulates described the criteria to be used to establish
scientifically the causality between disease and the
microorganism believed to be responsible. The isolation and
culture of the microorganism in question are here all-important.
This view had already been advanced in 1840 by Henle, the German
pathologist and anatomist (1809-1885).
Koch provided further evidence for this link by stating that the
injection of the resulting pure cultures (that is, cultures of
one bacterial strain) into healthy and susceptible experimental
animals must lead to characteristic syndromes in these animals.
Koch's postulates gained general acceptance in microbiology and
helped to lay the foundation for the intensive use of laboratory
animals. The animal assumed a key position within clinical and
experimental pathology, and the need for good animal "models"
increased when it was found that not every species is equally
sensitive to pathogenic microorganisms. For example, Koch used
mice, guinea pigs and rabbits as well as sheep for his work on
anthrax.
When it was difficult to find a suitable animal model, as was the
case with typhoid and cholera, the investigations stagnated. On
the other hand, rapid results were obtained in research on
diphtheria, when it was found that the guinea pig was a
relatively simple animal model.

2.3. The beginnings of vaccine development

The insight gained into the aetiology and course of infectious
diseases through animal experimentation* opened the way to the
discovery of an effective prophylactic and therapeutic solution
for a number of these diseases.
The real breakthrough came after Pasteur had published his
findings on fowl cholera. He discovered in 1880 that when
chickens were injected with old cultures of Pasteurella multocida
- the causative agent - very few clinical symptoms developed. A
subsequent injection of fresh virulent cultures into the same
animals had no adverse effects. He drew two fundamental
conclusions from this:
a. the virulence of germs can be attenuated by storing the
   culture for a some time, and
b. these cultures can be used to induce artificial immunity.
The vaccine against fowl cholera thus became the first
experimentally developed vaccine.
After the preparation of the fowl cholera vaccine, Pasteur used
the same approach in the development of an anthrax vaccine.

---

* In this context it is interesting to note that as early as 1798
  a smallpox vaccine was "developed" by Jenner, without much
  initial experimental research.

He succeeded in attenuating the causative microorganism by culturing it at 42oC. The scientific community was at first fairly sceptical about vaccination and to convince his critics Pasteur organized a public demonstration on 5 May 1881. The live attenuated anthrax vaccine was administered to 24 sheep, one goat and six cows. A similar group of animals served as controls. Pasteur then "challenged" (i.e. artificially infected) the animals with a virulent anthrax strain on 31 May. The controls died within the next few days, but all the vaccinated animals survived the experiment. The principle of challenge used by Pasteur for studying the immunogenic property of his vaccine can still be found in modern potency testing.

2.4. The rabies vaccine

Whereas the first vaccines were specifically intended for combatting diseases in animals, from 1881 onwards the focus was also on the development of human vaccines. Strangely enough the first success was achieved with a disease the pathogenesis of which was not fully understood. Between 1881 and 1885 Pasteur and his assistants Chamberlain (1851-1908) and Roux (1853-1933) studied canine madness (or rabies).

That a microorganism was responsible for the disease could be demonstrated by injecting saliva of infected animals or humans into rabbits. However, all attempts to "see" or culture the pathogenic microorganism failed. On the other hand, the microorganism did multiply in the cerebral and spinal cord tissues of animals which Pasteur had artificially infected by introducing it into their brain tissues. As a result, the incubation time, the period between infection and the first symptoms, was reduced from a few weeks to seven days. Next, Pasteur and his co-workers found that the virulence decreased when the material containing the virus was exposed to sterile air. The development of the first rabies vaccine was based on these observations. Rabbits were used for culturing the virus. After they died, their medulla oblongata (part of the central nervous system) was treated as described above and processed into an injectable product.

Vaccination of dogs with this product followed by inoculation (injection) of virulent virus proved its efficacy. The vaccine was first used in humans in 1885. A small boy, named Joseph Meister, was injected several times, starting 60 hours after having been bitten by a rabid dog. No clinical symptoms developed, and as a result of this success the method became widely used, as is illustrated by the fact that by 1889 over 20 institutes for rabies vaccination had been set up around the world. People jokingly called the vaccination method "tattooing" because as many as 20 injections were sometimes needed to confer effective protection.

Sheep, newborn rabbits or newborn mice were until recently used in the Netherlands and in many other countries for culturing the rabies virus. A problem with this in vivo produced vaccine was the sporadic occurrence of allergic encephalitis (inflammation of the brain tissue), a dreaded complication, which was largely solved (in the Netherlands in 1978) by the introduction of the vaccine produced by using cell cultures (dog kidney cells).

6

3. THE 20th CENTURY

Since Pasteur's pioneering work, immunization as a means of
combatting infectious diseases was taken up and extended by
several researchers. In all these cases the experimental animal
played an essential role, firstly in the development of a model
for clinico-pathological research, secondly in the selection of
vaccine strains and testing for immunogenic properties and,
finally, in the quality improvement and control of the vaccines.
Several sera and vaccines are listed below, together with the
name of the developer and the year of development/introduction.

Biological product	Developed by	Year
Smallpox vaccine	Jenner	1798
Fowl cholera vaccine	Pasteur	1880
Anthrax vaccine	Pasteur	1881
Rabies vaccine	Pasteur	1885
Swine fever vaccine	Salmon	1886
Diphtheria antiserum	Behring	1890
Tetanus antiserum	Kitasato	1890
Tuberculosis vaccine (BCG vaccine)	Calmette and Guérin	1906-21
Diphtheria vaccine	Ramon	1923
Pertussis vaccine	Madsen	1923
Leptospirosis (icterohaemorrhagiae serotype) vaccine	Dalling and Okell	1926
Tetanus vaccine	Ramon	1927
Mumps vaccine	Stokes	1945
Poliomyelitis vaccine	Salk and Sabin	1955-60
Measles vaccine	Katz	1958

It shows that, apart from smallpox and rabies vaccines, the
development of most viral vaccines did not begin until later.
This can be largely explained by the characteristics of the
microorganisms. Viruses only grow in cells so that, until the
introduction and the large-scale use of the tissue culture
technique, they had to be cultured in vivo (i.e. in live
animals). This was a complicating factor in the development of
vaccines, because the in vivo method implied that the production
capacity was limited. Furthermore, the vaccines also caused many
side effects. Landsteiner (1909), for example, succeeded in
inducing poliomyelitis experimentally in monkeys by introducing
the causative microorganism into their spinal cords, but attempts
to prepare a vaccine based on a spinal-cord suspension failed.
This limitation of the experimental animal in vaccine research
does not detract from the fundamental importance of the
experimental animal for this research. The place of animal
experiments in the development of diphtheria prophylaxis will be
discussed in detail in the next chapter.

4. REFERENCES

1. Zo doende 1986 (Animal experimentation in the Netherlands, Statistics 1986). Veterinary Public Health Inspectorate, Animal Experiments Department, Rijswijk, the Netherlands.
2. Müller, G. and Kiessig, R.: Einführung in die Versuchstierkunde, Band I: Allgemeine Versuchstierkunde (Introduction to the science of experimental animals. Vol. 1 General Aspects), Gustav Fischer Verlag, Jena, 1977
3. Bernard, C.: An introduction to the study of experimental medicine. Chapter III. Dover Publications. New York, 1957. (This is an English version of Bernard's work "Introduction à l'étude de la médecine expérimentale", originally published in France in 1865.)
4. Bernard, C.: Principes de médecine expérimentale (Principles of Experimental Medicine), Cahier Rouge, 1850-1867
5. Koch, R.: Die Aethiologie und die Bekämpfung der Tuberkulose (Aetiology and treatment of tuberculosis), 1884

CHAPTER 3: THE HISTORICAL ROLE OF ANIMAL EXPERIMENTS IN THE
DEVELOPMENT OF DIPHTHERIA PROPHYLAXIS

In several respects the experimental work carried out over the
decades to find a specific and reliable way of treating and
preventing diphtheria determined the use of laboratory animals in
the quality control of biological products in general. On the one
hand, diphtheria was one of the first diseases where experimental
animal research laid the foundation for combatting this disease
(1, 2). On the other hand, many common routine procedures such as
the determination of the efficacy of a vaccine and the use of a
standard vaccine arose from diphtheria research. Before
discussing the current method of vaccine production and control,
attention will therefore be paid to the history of diphtheria
prophylaxis and in particular to the significance of the animal
experiment in this.

1. INTRODUCTION

With a mortality rate of up to around 40%, diphtheria belonged to
one of the most feared epidemic diseases of childhood in the 19th
century (1). Infection, via the the respiratory tract, affected
mostly children aged 1 to 6 years, and it usually led to severe
breathing difficulties and damage to the internal organs (3).
There was no effective treatment; tracheostomy (incision of the
trachea) and bloodletting were regularly practised but were
seldom effective (4, 5).
The last epidemic in the Netherlands occurred between 1940 and
1948 and was caused by the poor living conditions and inadequate
medical provision during the war years (6). In this period there
was no specific treatment or prophylaxis available, probably
resulting in 220,000 cases of diphtheria with a mortality rate of
around 14% (6).
Diphtheria is now a rare disease in the Western countries. Only
363 cases were recorded in Europe in the period 1979-83 (7). This
sharp fall in both morbidity and mortality has, apart from
improved hygiene and diet, been ascribed especially to diphtheria
vaccines (1, 2). Laboratory animal research made an important
contribution to the development of these products, and data from
animal experiments are still used today in the quality control of
diphtheria vaccines. The link between diphtheria research and
animal experiment is consequently very firm, traditional and, in
terms of biology, cross-fertilising. New insights into the
treatment and prevention of diphtheria have influenced the way in
which animal experiments are performed, and vice versa. It has
yielded results which often served as a model for immunological
research in other fields.
For a closer consideration of the role of the experimental animal
in the history of diphtheria research, it is essential to
distinguish between three successive key areas:
a. clinico-pathological research to gain an insight into the
   development and course of the disease;
b. the development of methods of treatment and prophylaxis with
   diphtheria antiserum and diphtheria toxoid respectively;
c. the development of the quality control of these products.
Unlike areas a and b, area c is still evolving because new
scientific insights and concepts lead to a continual adjustment
of this quality control.

2. CLINICO-PATHOLOGICAL RESEARCH

Within the group of infectious diseases diphtheria was one of the
first disorders studied comprehensively. The initial impetus to
this was given in 1883 when Theobald Klebs isolated the
microorganism responsible (Corynebacterium diphtheriae) from the
throat of a young patient. However, Klebs did not provide
definitive proof of the causality. It was the German Friedrich
Loeffler who succeeded in doing so in 1884 (8). In accordance
with "Koch's Postulates" mentioned in the previous chapter, he
managed to induce in experimental animals the symptoms
characteristic of diphtheria (pseudomembranous inflammation of
the pharynx). Loeffler mentioned the use of pigeons, chickens,
rabbits and guinea pigs, which he had infected with pure cultures
of the Corynebacterium diphtheriae through lesions made in the
mucous membrane.
Although Loeffler could not provide evidence for this, he was one
of the first to suggest that the diphtheria bacillus was capable
of producing an exotoxin (i.e. an extracellular poison). He
believed that this might explain a clinico-pathological
phenomenon not yet understood at that time. It was known that
microorganisms could be cultured from the throat of patients who
had died from diphtheria but not from their internal organs,
despite the fact that the latter showed clear pathological
changes.
The French researchers Roux and Yersin used Loeffler's theory as
the basis for their study. They succeeded in preparing a sterile
filtrate from the diphtheria culture using porcelain filters.
Injection of this filtrate into various animal species
subsequently corroborated the theory proposed by Loeffler. The
finding made by Roux and Yersin in 1888 proved to be of crucial
importance. It paved the way to the search for a specific
antitoxin by means of immunology, entirely in accordance with the
scientific achievements of those days in this field. In the
concluding sentence of their article, Roux and Yersin had already
pointed more or less in this direction: "Is it possible to
habituate animals to the diphtheria poison and thus to induce in
them immunity against diphtheria?" (9).
Apart from furnishing proof of the existence of an exotoxin, the
article is also of historical importance for the reason that it
contains clear indications about the use of guinea pigs as the
most suitable species for diphtheria research, a view still held
today.

3. DIPHTHERIA PROPHYLAXIS

3.1. Development of the diphtheria antiserum
A biomedical-historical survey can easily create a wrong
impression. The succession of spectacular findings in the past
suggests that scientific research invariably leads to positive
results. However, nothing is further from the truth, as an
experiment performed by the German Emil von Behring illustrates.
This pupil of Koch was intrigued by the observation of Roux and
Yersin that some animal species have a natural immunity against
diphtheria. This gave Behring the idea - in itself quite
plausible - that these animals had "antibodies" against the
diphtheria toxin. However, attempts to transfer this immunity via
blood transfusion to diphtheria-susceptible animals where
unsuccessful: " ......we sought to obtain curative effects by
using the blood of animals which are naturally immune to

diphtheria. We have investigated the blood of mice, rats, dogs*, and later also the blood of all animals available to us in the laboratory and in the slaughterhouse, but did not obtain a positive result with any of these types of blood" (10). Despite this negative result, Behring pursued his original assumption, but he now used the blood of previously infected guinea pigs in subsequent experiments. His findings (" .... showed some indication of therapeutic results when we used the blood of diphtheria-infected guinea pigs") won him the Nobel prize in Medicine in 1901.

The first description in 1890 (11) of the diphtheria (and tetanus) antitoxin and of the therapeutic and prophylactic value of the blood serum of artificially infected guinea pigs (" ..... we have succeeded both in curing infected animals and in pretreating healthy ones in such a way that they later no longer fell ill with diphtheria or tetanus" (11)) meant a breakthrough in medicine. But not everyone shared this view. In 1891 the bacteriologist Fokker wrote in the Dutch Medical Journal: "Behring's statements, after the ones already published, will not satisfy many" (13).

However, for large-scale production of antitoxin - a prerequisite for human application - the guinea pig model was not adequate. Follow-on studies therefore focused on this quantitative aspect. An increase in production was achieved by collecting serum from infected dogs and sheep (10). Even flesh of infected slaughter animals (12) and goat's (14) and cow's milk (14) were tested in experimental animals for a possible protective effect. On the basis of research by Roux and Martin (15), the horse was eventually chosen in 1894 for producing the antiserum.

Within a few years, the diphtheria antiserum was used on a large scale for therapeutic purposes**.

It completely changed the previously hopeless treatment. A dangerously ill child could now be cured with one single injection (17). This result affected many people deeply and it also had its effect on the intensifying discussions in those days about the need for vivisection (18). The fact that experimental animal research had made the treatment of the feared disease possible convinced many of the value of this type of experimentation and undermined the criticism levelled at it (1). However, after the initial enthusiasm it was quite soon recognized that the antiserum also had its limitations. It was unsuitable for preventive purposes, it induced only short-lasting immunity following its administration, and occasionally caused side-effects, including anaphylactic reactions (19).

---

* Behring's supposition that dogs have natural immunity against diphtheria proved to be erroneous, as was demonstrated by the Dutchman Spronck by means of experiments in which he infected dogs and cats (12).

** On the whole, it found wider acceptance in the smaller than in the larger towns. Strauss wrote in 1890: "In the small towns where, compared to the large city, the lowest class is less brutalized, the situation is much more favourable and young patients come forward for early treatment" (16).

3.2. Toxin-antitoxin mixtures

At around the turn of the century Babes (20) and Smith (21) broke
new ground. They described the possibility of active immunization
with toxin-antitoxin mixtures. It was especially due to the
experimental animal work carried out by Behring (22) that this
form of immunization was brought to the notice of the general
public in 1913. However, it emerged that the method - having its
heyday between 1913 and 1925 - readily gave rise to anaphylactic
reactions (23), conferred a low degree of immunity and was
partcularly vulnerable to production errors. Numerous cases,
often fatal, of diphtheria intoxication resulting from the
presence of free toxin are known (24).
Because of these problems safety testing was introduced in the
twenties. Representative samples of the homogeneous final product
of each production, or vaccine, batch were examined for possible
toxic properties by administering it to susceptible animals. This
safety test is still part of the quality control in vaccine
production.

3.3. Diphtheria toxoid

The decline in the use of the toxin-antitoxin mixtures for active
immunization purposes was accelerated - apart from the
shortcomings mentioned above - by a finding of the French
researcher Ramon in 1923. He succeeded in detoxifying the
diphtheria toxin by heating and exposing it to formalin, with
preservation of its immunogenic properties. This final product
-called anatoxin by Ramon - was found to produce a high degree of
protective immunity in experimental animals (25). Before Ramon
other researchers had already attempted to detoxify the toxin
with iodine trichloride (von Behring (10), carbon disulphide
(Ehrlich (26) and formalin (Salkowski, 27; Löwenstein, 28;
Glenny, 29, 30) but none of these investigators could detoxify it
completely, as was shown in animal studies.
The effectiveness of Ramon's anatoxin was confirmed clinically
within a few months, albeit not without problems (31), and it
subsequently found worldwide application. The remedy did not
become known as anatoxin but as toxoid, a term introduced by
Ehrlich in 1898 (26). Since this toxoid - unlike toxin-anatoxin -
was prepared in vitro, the introduction of the toxoid meant that
the production of diphtheria vaccine no longer relied on
experimental animals.
In the years following Ramon's finding, the immunogenicity of the
toxoid could be augmented by the addition of adjuvants,
substances which, when added to the vaccine, increase immune
response. Ramon was one of the first to use the substance tapioca
for this purpose (32). However, the development of an abscess at
the site of injection was a major drawback and restricted its use
to experimental immunization in laboratory animals (33)! A number
of precipitating and adsorbing aluminium salts, such as $AlK(SO_4)_2$
(34), $AlPO_4$ (35) and $Al(OH)_3$ (36) had a much better adjuvant
effect. Extensive animal studies were conducted to elucidate the
mode of action of these adjuvants. Farago concluded, partly on
the basis of transplantation experiments in guinea pigs, that
there was a delay in the adsorption rate of the toxoid (37).
These adjuvated vaccines are still used for vaccination purposes
even today. Since the thirties, research - including on animals -
has mainly concentrated on improving the quality of the vaccine
as regards, for example, its purity.

4. QUALITY CONTROL

4.1. Historical development

The current sera and vaccines belong to the class of biological products. This origin determines for a large part the extent of quality control. The reason is that differences may arise in consecutive batches because several variables influence the production process. Each batch must therefore be examined.
The need for such an examination had already emerged very early in the development of sera and vaccines, as is illustrated by a remark made by Behring about the diphtheria antiserum: " ....
Irrespective of how the immunization may have been achieved and what animals were used, be it guinea pigs, rabbits or sheep, the outcome regarding the protective and healing effects of the blood of the immunized animals was qualitatively always the same; it differed only quantitatively (10)".
However, this quantitative difference, which in 1893 was to some extent glossed over by Behring, posed problems in the human application of the diphtheria antiserum. The therapeutic effect could differ from batch to batch, from nil to excellent. This made the development of some kind of efficacy assay an absolute necessity. The efficacy, or potency, assay is even today still one of the main pillars of the control of sera and vaccines, relying first and foremost on animal tests.
The German Paul Ehrlich was the pioneer in the field of potency testing. He assumed that the degree of immunization of an antiserum-producing animal is a measure for the effectiveness of the product. For that purpose, he used a figure corresponding to that multiple of the minimum lethal dose of diphtheria toxin that was only just tolerated by the immunized animals. In practice, however, this method was found to have numerous drawbacks, one of the major ones being that it could not be used in large antiserum-producing animals.
In 1892, Behring and Wernicke (10) introduced an indirect assay method for efficacy based on the principle of passive protection. Serial dilutions of the serum of immunized animals were injected into a group of guinea pigs. Twelve hours later, each animal received a quantity of diphtheria broth culture (later replaced with toxin), the strength of which was just sufficient to kill non-immunized animals within 4 days. As a criterion for determining the efficacy, Behring and Wernicke chose that serum dilution which only just protected animals against death, but not against clinical and macroscopic diphtheria signs and symptoms. Neither did this method yield reliable results; too many variables, such as the variation in the sensitivity of the individual animals and differences in the virulence of the toxin, influenced the determination.

4.2. The French and German methods

In France, Roux and his associates developed an assay in 1894 which became known as the French method (15, 38). The theoretical basis of this method was novel insofar that Roux made a fundamental distinction between the preventive potency (pouvour prréventif) and the curative potency (pouvoir curatif) of the antiserum. There was an animal model for both these aspects of the potency. The determination of the "pouvoir curatif" was a variant on von Behring's method. The "pouvoir préventif" was determined by administering serum dilutions to guinea pigs 6 hours after injection of diphtheria toxin.

There was a rapid succession of ideas about the design of the
potency test in the 1890s. Each new version had to be validated
and - since each method was based on an animal model - required
the necessary animals. The impression is sometimes created that
few test animals were used at the end of the last century;
however, for diphtheria research alone, thousands of animals must
have been sacrificed each year, mainly in France and Germany.
A few years after Roux, Ehrlich (1897) described an assay method
which went down in history as the German method (39). Unlike the
previous methods in common use, Ehrlich mixed serial dilutions of
antiserum with a constant amount of diphtheria toxin prior to
their injection into animals. The resulting toxin-antitoxin
mixtures varied in composition and, depending on the quantity of
antiserum, ranged from fully neutralized toxin to free toxin. His
finding that under certain conditions (for example, under vacuum)
the protective power of the antiserum was not lost, also broke
new ground.
To eliminate the influence of such variables as the variation in
sensitivity of the individual animals and differences in
virulence, Ehrlich decided to use the toxin-neutralizing power of
a particular antiserum as a unit for determination of the potency
of an unknown antiserum. He employed an arbitrary antiserum of
known potency as a standard and thereby introduced into the
control of human biological products the regular use of standard
preparations as a unit of measure. The use of a standard
preparation still is an integral part of the potency testing of
vaccines.
By the German method, the value of an unknown antiserum is
determined by the L+ dose or the L_0 dose of both the antiserum
being tested and the standard antiserum. The L+ dose is the
smallest amount of diphtheria toxin which, when mixed with one
international unit (I.U.) of diphtheria antitoxin before being
injected subcutaneously, will kill a 250-gram guinea pig on day
four following injection. The L_0 dose is the amount of diphtheria
toxin which causes clinical symptoms under similar conditions. By
comparing the value found for the unknown antiserum with the
value for the standard serum, the relative potency of the former
can be calculated in International Units.
In the early stage in particular, there were heated debates about
the pros and cons of the French and German methods, often
corroborated by the debaters' own experimental (animal) research
(40-43). Because of its greater reliability the German method was
quite unanimously chosen and it found worldwide application
accordingly.
Until the onset of World War I, the Ehrlich Institute in
Frankfurt guaranteed the provision of the standard serum. After
1914, this function, as a result of the changed international
relations, was partly taken over by an institute in Washington
DC, USA. Because of the use of different standard sera it became
no longer possible to intercompare the various antisera. In 1922,
the State Serum Institute in Copenhagen was therefore chosen by
the Committee on diphtheria and tetanus antisera of the League of
Nations to monitor the uniformity of the standard sera being
used.
But the German method, of course, also had its critics. In 1913,
Krause and Bacher (44) concluded after extensive animal studies,
based on the methods then in common use, that there was no
correlation between the therapeutic effect and the number of
International Units of an antiserum, as calculated by the German
method. This view was endorsed by Ramon (45).

In the same article of 1923 Ramon also introduced a method which can perhaps be regarded as one of the first in vitro techniques in the quality control of vaccines. This method is known as Limes flocculation, Lf test or Ramon flocculation. It makes it possible to measure the amount of antitoxin or toxin (and later also toxoid) in a simple manner. Tubes with constant amounts of toxoid are mixed with variable amounts of standard serum and incubated at 45oC. The first tube which shows flocculation contains neither excess of antitoxin nor excess of toxoid, so the amount of antitoxin expressed in Lf equivalents is equal to the amount of toxoid expressed in Lf.

The Lf method was briefly the official potency assay. It soon became clear that although the Lf method was eminently suitable for determining the amount of antigen (or antibody) present, it gave no indication of the quality (read immunogenicity) of the product, that is, two products having the same flocculation value could nevertheless differ widely in efficacy (2, 3, 37, 46, 47). The method consequently lost its importance as a final control test, but it remained in use for making a rapid intermediate assessment of the product during the so-called in-process control.

4.3. The influence of statistics

Since the 1930s there has been a train of developments in diphtheria research which proved to be important as regards the use of experimental animals. For example, achievements made in experimental pharmacology, in particular those relating to the statistical processing of experimental data, were introduced into the quality control of vaccines.

At the same time, there was far-reaching internationalization of regulations in the field of quality control. These aspects are most evident in potency testing because, as a result of the development of the new toxoid vaccines, there was a growing need for an accurate assay for these products.

The methods used until then could scarcely be described as accurate. Broadly, there were two versions (3), one based on the determination of the amount of antitoxin in the serum of immunized guinea pigs, the other on immunization of a group of guinea pigs, followed by a challenge with diphtheria toxin.

Through research many variables were recognized which - apart from the vaccine dose - could affect the outcome of a potency assay. These external variables could in part be related to experimental conditions such as the apparatus, personnel, or methodology used, but such factors as diet, season (48) and the animal strain could also influence the immune response of the animals. This could result in widely different values for one and the same vaccine.

For example, in a large-scale study in guinea pigs, Prigge (2) found a difference of a factor of 32,000, between the amount of toxoid required to protect the best immunizable and the least immunizable animal. That such conditions become less relevant when the relative potency of an unknown product is read against a standard preparation of known strength has been known since the time of Ehrlich's fundamental research quoted above.

In 1931, the German researcher Prigge pressed for the development of a standard toxoid to be used internationally (47). However, it was not until December 1951 that the WHO Expert Committee on Biological Standardization designated as the standard vaccine a toxoid produced for this purpose by the National Institutes of Health (Bethesda, USA) (50, 51). The State Serum Institute in

Copenhagen assumed a central position in monitoring the quality
of the WHO standard vaccine.

4.4. The "Kollektivversuch" or "group test"

The use of a standard vaccine as a reference is only a partial
solution to the problem of reproducibility in potency testing.
There remains the variation in the sensitivity of the individual
experimental animals to the action of a vaccine, which can give
rise to large differences in the final result of the assay (2, 3,
49, 52). It was Prigge who, on the basis of research using large
groups of guinea pigs, concluded that in a large animal
population this individual sensitivity obeys a binomial
distribution (47). This led him to recommend in 1937 that in
potency testing not the then-accepted principle of using one or a
few animals per dose, the so-called "einfachen Reihenversuch", be
applied, but that for each dose a group of animals be taken as a
representative sample of the animal population, the so-called
"Kollektivversuch".

To some extent, Prigge's "Kollektivversuch" concept had its
origin in experimental pharmacology, where great importance was
attached to the statistical processing of a bioassay. This
discipline also created such concepts as the ED50* and the 95%
confidence interval, now commonly used in immunology.

To overcome the individual variation mentioned above, the ED50
test was introduced.

This test is derived from the LD50 test which was originally
developed by Trevan (53) in 1927. LD50 stands for "lethal dose-50
per cent" and it indicates the dose of a substance which will
kill half of a group of animals. For statistical reasons the LD50
is easier to estimate accurately than the minimum lethal dose or
the maximum non-lethal dose. Trevan's concept of LD50 was thus a
valuable contribution to the standardization of biological
products.

The principle of the 95% confidence interval is based on the
finding that even in a group test the calculation involves a
certain error. The confidence interval, which is determined
statistically, gives numerically an idea of this error (54). The
larger the number of animals used for a determination, the
smaller the error in this determination and the narrower the
confidence interval. Trevan (53) considered the ideal number of
animals for a potency test to be 30 for each vaccine dilution.

In an article published in 1939 Prigge (2) arrived at a concrete
proposal for the potency test, based on the knowledge available:
"Several groups of guinea pigs are injected with increasing
amounts of antigen, ranging from a dose that is ineffective in
all animals (0%) to a dose that is effective in all (100%). (Each
animal receives only one antigen injection). Next, the percentage
of animals which is protected when injected with varying doses of
toxin is determined. When the percentage of protected animals is
plotted against the antigen dose, an S-shaped dose-response curve
or "efficacy curve" is obtained of the vaccine being tested" (2,
p. 9).

---

* ED stands for effective dose, and is the amount of vaccine
  which, following challenge of the animals with the virulent
  microorganisms (or toxin), produces protection in 50% of the
  population.

"The effectiveness of a diphtheria vaccine is now measured by determining that dose with the same effect as a reference dose of the standard preparation, under the same external conditions" (2, p. 13).
"A proper 'determination' of the efficacy is only possible when the 'efficacy curves' run parallel" (2, p. 13).
This design - also called parallel-line bioassay - is very similar to the assay we use today, not only for the diphtheria toxoid but also for several other inactivated vaccine products (including tetanus, whooping cough and rabies vaccines). The model described by Prigge has since been modified, for example, as regards the number of vaccine dilutions. Thus, before 1940 a 2-point assay was in force in Germany, requiring 125 animals for each dilution both of the test vaccine and of the reference vaccine (55). A qualitative assay, which was a legal requirement in the Netherlands in the late forties, was based on a course of injections with diphtheria toxoid into each of 12 guinea pigs, followed by a challenge with toxin. At least 9 animals should survive the experiment (56). A decade later the parallel-line assay was revived in the form of a 6-point assay, that is, the potency is determined by using 3 dilutions of the test vaccine and 3 dilutions of the reference vaccine. Initially, the number of animals was 30 for each dilution (57). At present, 16 guinea pigs are needed per dilution, thus making a total of 96 animals (58).

5. RECENT DEVELOPMENTS

Numerous new approaches to diphtheria vaccine control have since been evaluated, including several in vitro methods such as an enzyme-linked immunosorbent assay (ELISA) and haemagglutination. To date, however, the degree of correlation between these new methods and the in vivo test is still unsatisfactory (59). This is not true of an in vivo alternative based on an intradermal challenge (60). In this assay, groups of guinea pigs are vaccinated with various dilutions of the reference preparation and of the test vaccine. After a given immunization period the animals are challenged intracutaneously with different doses of diphtheria toxin, each animal receiving 5 doses. Non-neutralized toxin causes a characteristic redness of the skin (erythema), which can be used instead of death to calculate the potency of the vaccine being tested. The advantages of this method - included in the European Pharmacopoeia as an alternative to the lethal potency test (61) - are the replacement of the lethal challenge with an intradermal challenge (i.e. a more human test) and the reduction of the number of animals required. On the other hand, disadvantages include the subjectivity of the assessment criteria and the labour intensiveness of this method.
A methodology (the mouse model) developed by Kreeftenberg appears to be particularly promising (62, 63). The efficacy is no longer determined by means of a lethal or intradermal challenge but by serum titration in Vero cells, a non-tumourigenic cell line, originally derived from kidney cells of an African green monkey (Cercopithecus aethiops). Briefly, the principle of this method is based on vaccination of two sets of four groups of 8 mice each, with dilutions of the reference preparation and the vaccine being tested, respectively. After an immunization period of 5 weeks the animals are bled under anaesthesia. Next, the content of toxin-neutralizing antibodies in the blood is determined by titration of serum dilutions with constant amounts of toxin using

Vero cells (the criterion being a cytopathological effect on the Vero cells).

This model which was recently introduced in the WHO guidelines (64) contributes to a desired reduction and refinement of animal experiments in two ways. First, refinement is achieved through the replacement of the distress-causing challenge by a combined bleeding and euthanasia procedure under anaesthesia. Secondly, the number of animals required per test can be reduced considerably because more information is obtained from each animal. Actually, the latter may also be realized on other grounds. Research in Canada as well as in England and the Netherlands has shown that the number of animals required for potency testing can be cut down drastically (up to 50%) if products of consistent high quality can be made, as is indeed the case with the diphtheria and tetanus vaccines (65).

Two other animal tests playing a role in diphtheria vaccine control have not been discussed here. They are the specific-toxicity test and the abnormal-toxicity test (see Chapter 4), but neither has undergone modification after its introduction into routine testing. An in vitro alternative to the specific-toxicity test has recently been reported (65). It is currently being validated and will be discussed later (see Chapter 8, 4.3.).

In general, since the introduction of the diphtheria antiserum in 1890, millions of laboratory animals have been required for both the development of newer, better products and the routine control of existing preparations. It is partly because of experimental animal studies that a diphtheria toxoid is now available which is both effective and safe. This in turn may lead to a considerable reduction in the number of animals required in this field.

6. REFERENCES

1. Turner, J.: Reckoning with the beast. The Johns Hopkins University Press, Baltimore (1980), p. 115, ISBN 0-8018-2399-4.
2. Prigge, R.: Diphtherie-Schutzimpfungen mit hochactiven Impfstof. (Diphtheria vaccination with highly active vaccines.) Ergebnisse der Hygiene, (1939), 22, 1-63.
3. Ramshorst, J.D. van and Ehrengut, E.: Diphtherieschutzimpfung (Diphtheria vaccination, in the book entitled Handbuch der Schutzimpfungen (Vaccination Manual) by Herrlich, A., (1965), p. 394, Springer Verlag, Berlin.
4. Parish, H.J.: A history of immunization. E and S Livingstone Ltd., Edinburgh/London, 1965.
5. Guye.: Ned. Tijdschrift v. Geneeskunde (1889), II, 13, p.435.
6. Hoogendoorn, D.: Statistisch onderzoek naar de uitkomsten der inentingen tegen difterie. (Statistical examination of the results of diphtheria vaccination.) Ned. Tijdschr. Geneeskd. (1949), 93, III, 37, 3153-62.
7. Kwantes, W.: Diphtheria in Europe, J. Hyg. Camb. (1984), 93, 433-437.
8. Loeffler, M.: Untersuchung über die Bedeutung der Microorganismen für die Entstehung der Diphtherie beim Menschen, bei der Taube and beim Kalbe. (The role of microorganisms in the causation of diphtheria in man, pigeons and calves.) Mitteilungen aus den Kaiserl. Gesundheitsamte, Vol. II, (1884), p. 421.
9. Roux, E. and Yersin, A.: Contribution à l'étude de la diphthérie. (Contribution to the study of diphtheria.)Annales de l'Institut Pasteur, (1888), 2, 12, 629-661.
10. Behring, E. von and Wernicke: Uber Immunisierung und Heilung von Versuchstieren bei der Diphtherie. (Immunisation and cure of experimental animals with respect to diphtheria.) Zeitschrift für Hygiëne, (1892), 12, 10-44.
11. Behring, E. von and Kitasato: Uber das Zustandekommen der Diphtherie-Immunität und der Tetanus-Immunität bei Tieren. (Production of diphtheria immunity and tetanus immunity in animals.) Deutsche Medizinische Wochenschrift, (1890), 49, 113.
12. Wernicke: Ein experimenteller beitrag zur kenntnis des Löffler-schen Diphtheriebacillus und zur "Blutserumtherapie". (Experimental work on Loeffler's dipththeria bacillus and blood serum therapy.) Archiv. für Hygiene, (1893), XVIII, 193-250.
13. Fokker: Ned. Tijdschr. Geneesk., (1891), I, 1, p. 19.
14. Ehrlich, P. and Wassermann, A.: Uber die Gewinnung der Diphtherie-Antitoxine aus Blutserum und Milch immunisierter Tiere. (Preparation of diphtheria from the serum and milk of immunized animals.) Zeitschr. für Hygiene, (1894), 18, 239-251.
15. Roux, M.E. and Martin, M.L.: Contribution à l'étude de la Diphthérie. (Contribution to the study of diphtheria.) Annales de l'Institut Pasteur, (1894), 8, 9, 609.
16. Strauss, M.: De serum-therapie der Diphtherie. (Serum therapy of diphtheria.) Ned. Tijdschr. Geneesk. (1899), I, 6, 197-209.
17. Bierens de Haan, J.C.: De uitkomsten der serumbehandeling van diptherie aan het Leidsche ziekenhuis van 1894-1899. (Results of diphtheria serum treatment in the Leiden Hospital, 1894-99.) Ned. Tijdschr. Geneeskd. (1899), II, 289-297.

18. Virchow, R.: An address on the value of pathological experiments, The British Medical Journal, (1881), 198-204.
19. Anonymus: Klinische und therapeutische Mitteilungen. (Clinical and therapeutic communications.) Wiener Klinische Wochenschrift, (1895), 10, 190.
20. Babes, V.: Bull, Acad. Méd. (Paris), (1895), 34, 216.
21. Smith, T.: Active immunity produced by so-called balanced or neutral mixtures of diphtheria toxin and antitoxin. J. Exp. Med. (1909), 102, 1288-1289.
22. Behring, E. von: Uber ein neues Diphtherieschutzmittel. (A new anti-diphtheria agent.) Deutsche Medizinische Wochenschrift, (1913), 39, 19, 873-876.
23. Otto, R. and Blumenthal, G.: Weitere tierexperimentelle Beitrage zur aktiven Immunisierung gegen Diphtherie. (Further animal experiments concerning active immunization against diphtheria.) Zeitsch. für Hygiene, (1930), 111, 380.
24. Wilson, G.S.: The Hazards of Immunization, The Athlone Press (1969).
25. Ramon, G.: Sur le pouvoir floculant et sur les propriétés immunisantes d'une diphthérique rendue anatoxique (anatoxine). (Flocculating activity and immunizing properties of a diphtheria anatoxin.) C.R. Acad. Sci. (1923), 177, 1338-1342.
26. Ehrlich, P.: Klin. Jahrbuch (1898), 6, 299.
27. Salkowski, E.: Uber die Wirkung der Antiseptica auf Toxine. (Effect of antiseptics on toxins.) Berl. Klin. Wschr. (1898), 35, 545-549.
28. Löwenstein, E. and Eisler, R. von: über den Einfluss des Formaldehyd auf Blutserum. (Effect of formaldehyde on blood serum.) Zentralb. für Bakt. Origin. (1912), 261-281.
29. Glenny, A.T. and Hopkins, B.E.: Diphtheria toxoid as an immunizing agent. Brit. J. Exp. Pathol. (1923), 4, 283-288.
30. Glenny, A.T. and Südmersen: Notes on the production of immunity to diphtheria toxin. J. of Hyg. (1921), 20, 184.
31. Lévy, F.M.: The fiftieth anniversary of diphtheria and tetanus immunization. Preventive Medicine, (1975), 4, 226-237.
32. Ramon, G.: Sur la production de l'antitoxine diphtérique. (Production of diphtheria antitoxin.) C.R. Acad. Sci. (Paris). (1925), 93, 506.
33. Günther, O.: Antagonism and synergy of antigens. Bull. Wld. Hlth. Org. (1955), 13, 479-489.
34. Glenny, A.T.: J. Path. Bact. (1926), 29, 38.
35. Holt, L.B. and Bousfeld, G.: Brit. Med. J. (1949), 1, 695.
36. Schmidt, S. and Hansen: Uber die Reinigung und konzentrierung von Diphtherie-toxin und Diphtherie-anatoxin mit besonderem Hinblick auf die aktive Immunisierung von Menschen. (Purification and concentration of diphtheria toxin and anatoxin with special reference to active immunization in man.) Biochem. Z. (1930), 228, 263.
37. Farago, F.: Uber das Schicksal und die Wirksamkeit des Anatoxin Präzipitatdepots im Organismus. (Fate and activityof the anatoxin precipitate depot in the body.) Zeitschr.Immun. Forsch. (1935), 86, 191-204.
38. Roux, M.E., Martin, M.L. and Chaillou, P.: Trois cents cas de diphtérie par le serum antidiphthérique. (300 Cases of diphtheria caused by anti-diphtheria serum.) Annales de l'Institut Pasteur, (1894), VIII, 9, 640-667.

39. Ehrlich, P.: Die Wehrtbemessung des Diphtherieheilserums und deren theoretische Grundlage. (Assessing the potency of the diphtheria serum and its theoretical foundations) Klin. Jahrbuch, (1897), Vol. VI, 299.

40. Marx: Experimentelle Untersuchungen über die Beziehung zwischen den Gehalt an Immunitätseinheiten und dem schützenden und heilenden Werth der Diphtherieheilsera. (Experimental investigation of the connection between the level of immunity units and the protective and therapeutic activity of diphtheria sera.) Zeitschr. für Hygiene, (1901), 38, 372-285.

41. Madsen, Th.: Uber Messung der Stärke des antidiphtherischen Serums. (Determination of the activity of anti-diphtheria serum.) Zeitschr. für Hygiene, (1897), 24, 425-443.

42. Dreyer, G. and Madsen, Th.: Über Immunisierung mit den Toxonen des Diphtheriegiftes. (Immunization with the toxoids of the diphtheria toxin.) Zeitschr. für Hygiene, (1901), 37, 250-267.

43. Prausnitz, C.: III Die Standardisierung von Heilseren, serologischen Reaktionen und Impfstoffen. (Standardizing antitoxins, serological reactions and vaccines. Part III.) Ergebnisse der Immunitätsforschung, (1929), 10, 271-332.

44. Krause, R. and Backer, S.: Zbl. Bakt., I Abt. Ref. Suppl. (1913), 57, 106.

45. Ramon, G.: La floculation dans les mélanges de toxine et de sérum antidiphtérique. (Flocculation in mixtures of antidiphtheria serum and toxin.) Annales de l'Institut Pasteur, (1923), 37, 12, 1001-1011.

46. Glenny, A.T. and Barr, M.: Alum-toxoid precipitates as antigens. Journ. of Path., (1931), 34, 118-119.

47. Prigge, R.: Experimentelle Untersuchungen über die Wirksamkeit von Diphtherie Impfstoffen. (Experimental investigations of the activity of diphtheria vaccines.) Deutsch. Med. Wochenschr., (1937), 39, 1478-1482.

48. Madsen, Th. and Schmidt, S.: Seasonal variation in the susceptibility of laboratory animals to diphtheria toxin. Acta Soc. Medic Fenn. Duodecim, Ser. A. 15, (1932); 15.

49. Prigge, R.: Theorie und Methodik der Antigenmessung. (Theory and method of antigen determination.) Zeitschr. für Hygiene, (1937), 119, 186-192.

50. Greenberg, L.: International standardization of diphtheria toxoids. Bull. Wld. Hlth. Org., (1953), 9, 829-836.

51. World Health Organization, Expert Committee on Biological Standardization. (1952), Wld. Hlth. Org. Tech. Rep. Ser., 56, 4, 5.

52. Bonin, O.: Einige Grundlagen der Prüfung von Biologische Produkten. (Basis of testing biological products.) In the book entitled Handbuch der Schutzimpfungen (Vaccination Manual). Herrlich, A., (1965), p. 53, Springer Verlag, Berlin.

53. Trevan, J.W.: The error of determination of toxicity. Proc. Roy. Soc. (London), (1927), 101B, 483-514.

54. Trevan, J.W.: A statistical note on the testing of anti-dysentry sera. Journ. of Path., (1929), Vol. 32, 127-135.

55. Vorschriften für die Staatl, Prüfung der Impfstoffe zur aktiven Schutzimpfung gegen Diphtherie. (Instructions for the official testing of vaccines intended for active immunization against diphtheria.) Issued by the German Ministry of Internal Affairs, Ministerialbl. f.d. Innere Verwaltung (1935), 52, p. 1525.

22

56. Noordam, A.L. et al.: De nieuwe diphtherie-entstof, PT. (The new diphtheria vaccine called PT.) Ned. Tijdschr. Geneesk. (1949), 93, 48, 4014-1419.
57. Bonebakker, A. et al.: Vaccinatie tegen infectieziekten. (Vaccination against infectious diseases.) Stafleu's Wetenschappelijke Uitgeversmaatschappij N.V., Leiden (1965).
58. W.H.O.-Technical Report Series 638 (1979).
59. Hardegree, M.C.: WHO Ad Hoc Meeting: Potency testing of toxoids, Geneva, Dec. 12-14, 1983.
60. Knight, P.A.: A consideration of some methods by which the cost of potency assays for diphtheria and tetanus vaccines might be reduced. Develop. Biol. Standard. (1978), 41, 67-72.
61. European Pharmacopoeia, (Suppl. Vol. III (1977)).
62. Kreeftenberg, J.G. et al.: A mouse model to estimate the potency of the diphtheria component in combined vaccines, Symposium IABS, April 1985, London. Develop. Biol. Standard (1986), 64, 21-24.
63. Kreeftenberg, J.G. et al.: An investigation of a mouse model to estimate the potency of the diphtheria component in vaccines. Journ. Biol. Standard. (1985), 13, 229-234.
64. W.H.O.-Technical Report Series 760 (1987).
65. Kreeftenberg, J.G.: Report of an informal meeting about alternative methods for the potency control of the diphtheria and tetanus components in vaccines, Bilthoven, December 1985. Develop. Biol. Standard. (1986), 65, 261-266.
66. Abreo, C.B. and Stainer, D.W.: A tissue culture assay for diphtheria toxicity testing. Symposium IABS, April 1985, London. Develop. Biol. Standard. (1986), 64, 33-37.

CHAPTER 4: VACCINE DEVELOPMENT AND PRODUCTION

Since the beginning of this century the major infectious diseases
no longer pose a threat to man and (domesticated) animals in the
Western countries. This achievement can be largely ascribed to
mass active immunization (1, 2, 3). There are now many vaccines
available for both human and veterinary use. The previous
chapters showed that animal experiments have been (and still are)
of vital importance in the development and production of these
vaccines. To establish what role animal experiments play in
current vaccine research, several aspects of this research
relevant to the use of experimental animals will be considered in
the following paragraphs, viz. vaccine development, production
and control as well as national and international guidelines and
Good Manufacturing Practice (GMP).

1. DEVELOPMENT

The development of new products is an important part of vaccine
research. Until recently, attention was mainly focussed on
bacterial and viral diseases. However, scientific progress opens
up new horizons. Successes have also been reported in the past
few years in the field of protozoal (4) and parasitic (5)
diseases.
In general, it is especially socio-economic, medical and/or
political rather than academic considerations that underlie the
development of a new product. As a result, vaccine development
occupies a central position in society, as exemplified by the
commitment to develop vaccines against such diseases as AIDS and
African swine fever.
The development of a vaccine generally requires extensive
experimental animal research, although this need not always be
the case. A relevant animal model for pathological-
microbiological research is here of paramount importance. The
results of such research often form the starting point for the
development of a new vaccine. Animal experiments are required in
selecting the starting material (bacterial or viral strain), with
special attention to immunogenicity, toxic properties and
potential for inactivation or attenuation (i.e. reducing the
virulence of the microorganisms), for example, by passage in
cells or animals.
They are also needed to establish such factors as the stability
and formulation (composition) of the vaccine, and the mode and
frequency of administration. Human field trials play an important
role in the last stage of human vaccine development.
On the basis of the results the new vaccine can be submitted to
the proper authorities for registration.
Research into new and unconventional techniques is now the focus
of attention in immunology. The subunit vaccines (for example
purified (Sato's) pertussis vaccine) and the DNA recombinant
vaccines (for example an E. coli vaccine) now find application,
albeit still on a modest and often experimental scale. Vaccines
prepared according to different production techniques, such as
synthetic peptide vaccines and anti-idiotype vaccines are still
in an experimental stage. The development work for these
vaccines, too, requires animal models to answer questions about
quality aspects of products thus obtained.

The animal experiments performed as part of the development of new vaccines or new production techniques are generally of a fundamental nature and vary widely in design. Furthermore, accessibility to the results of these animal studies is limited when the development of new products is confidential. It is therefore difficult to discuss specific ways of reducing or refining the use of animals in this field. Nevertheless, guidelines on routine batch controls are usually drawn up on the basis of these animal experiments. Limitation (in the sense of reducing the number of animals) or refinement of animal research in the development stage can consequently have an enhanced effect on the use of animals in the quality control of vaccine batches. This observation does not however reject the proposition that good and extensive developmental research is of vital importance for quality control research.

2. PRODUCTION

The aim of vaccination is to induce specific protection against a certain infectious disease in the vaccinee. This protection - based on humoral (antibodies) or cellular immunity - results from the administration of a modified form of the microorganism (or components thereof) responsible for the disease. The part of the microorganism that is capable of inducing a specific immune response is called the antigen.
Almost all the existing vaccines have a bacterial or viral origin, the modification usally being the result of inactivation or attenuation of the virulent microorganism or components thereof. Occasionally non-virulent strains are used. The aim of the production process is to supply a high-quality product, i.e. where long-term specific immunity develops after its administration without serious adverse reactions. The conventional production techniques still in common use for bacterial and viral vaccines briefly are described below.

2.1. Bacterial vaccines
The first step in the production of bacterial vaccines is the selection of the starting material, the bacterial strain. As a rule, this bacterial strain is used for production purposes for many years. To that end, the strain is either stored in liquid nitrogen or is freeze-dried (and is called "seed-lot"). The various manufacturers prepare a so-called "working seed lot" from microorganisms of the seed lot. These microorganisms are also stored in liquid nitrogen or in the freeze-dried state, thus ensuring a stable starting material. For each production batch, microorganisms from the working seed lot are cultured in liquid or on solid media under specified conditions. After a given period the bacterial culture or the toxin-containing culture fluid can be harvested, This is referred to as the "crude vaccine bulk". Since this bulk is usually contaminated with bacterial secretions and/or components of the nutrient medium and has, moreover, a low antigen concentration, the next step in the production process consists of purification and concentration. Inactivation of the product (at least in the case of killed vaccines) also takes place at this stage, commonly with formalin, and an adjuvant may be added (see Chapter 3, 3.3).
The product thus obtained is referred to as "purified bulk" or "purified toxoid".
For the preparation of combined vaccines (such as, for example, the DPT-polio vaccine against diphtheria, pertussis, tetanus and

poliomyelitis) the other vaccine components are now added and the final product (the so-called final bulk) is then divided into a number of batches.

The last step in the production process is filling ampoules with suitable doses of the batch (the so-called final lot), followed by freeze-drying, if required.

2.2. Virus vaccines

The production of viral vaccines is broadly similar to that of the bacterial vaccines. It also involves a seed lot (seed virus), purification, concentration, packaging, followed by freeze-drying of most vaccines to increase shelf-life.

However, there are also clear differences. Another terminology is sometimes used, for example, virus suspension instead of bulk. In addition, virus propagation, unlike bacterial propagation, occurs in cells of animal or human origin. Accordingly, in vivo culturing methods had to be used in the past. Examples include the production of the smallpox virus on the skin of calves, or the rabies virus in the brains of mice, rabbits, sheep or goats, and of the Gumboro virus in the bursa of chickens.

However, since the fundamental research of Enders in 1949 into the use of primary cell cultures* for growing the polio virus (6) and that of Goodpasture in 1931 into the application of embryonated hen's eggs, virus vaccines have largely been produced using in vitro methods.

However, it may seem somewhat contradictory, given the above, to call the current tissue culture methods for the virus vaccines convential. After all advances in this field have been made only very recently. The monolayer cultures** of primary cells which were originally used on a large scale can increasingly be replaced by subcultured cells (e.g. tertiary kidney cell cultures in the case of polio), diploid cell strains or even cell lines (8).

In addition, the introduction of the microcarrier technique made it possible to increase the virus yield. Until recently, scale-up of production was hampered by technical and spatial limitations. Apart from a few exceptions, cells can multiply only after adhering to a suitable carrier, for which the bottoms of Povitsky flasks were initially used. The microcarrier technique is based on the use of DEAE Sephadex beads to which the cells can adhere, providing a surface area 5-10 times larger than with the Povitsky method. An additional advantage of the microcarrier system is that it produces a very homogeneous virus suspension under standardizable production conditions.

In general, the microcarrier technique is used only for those vaccine products which require large volumes of virus suspension, that is, for the inactivated viral vaccines against polio and rabies (9). Since with live vaccines, such as mumps, polio (oral), measles, canine distemper and avian infectious bronchitis, the virus will continue to multiply in the body of

---

*   Primary cells are directly derived from healthy human or animal tissues which are cultured in vitro as separate cells after their release from the tissue by trypsinization or by mechanical means (7).

** In a monolayer the cells have grown into a single, confluent layer by adhering to an artificial substrate.

the vaccinee after administration, a smaller amount of virus is
usually required. No description of the production process of
bacterial and viral vaccines can be complete without mentioning
the importance of consistency, that is, the fact that the final
products are always of good, uniform quality. To obtain such
consistency, the factors that may influence the production
process and quality testing must be controllable. Also, the
production process and quality control must be monitored to
ensure that they proceed as required. This is referred to as
"Quality Assurance". The importance of consistency is directly
related to the purpose of this report, for the quality of the
product is always connected with the nature, extent and frequency
of animal experiments.

3. VACCINE PRODUCTION IN THE NETHERLANDS

Within the scope of this book it is impossible to evaluate all
the vaccines produced in the world. Therefore, only the products
made in the Netherlands will be discussed as well as the live,
attenuated polio vaccine.
Vaccines are produced in seven centres in the Netherlands. Two
centres produce only human vaccines, four centres only veterinary
vaccines and one centre makes both veterinary and (one) human
vaccines. As regards the human vaccines, the Netherlands occupies
a unique position internationally because they are, with the
exception of the influenza and hepatitis B vaccines, produced by
government order.
The human and veterinary vaccines surveyed for this project are
given in Table 1.

Table 1: SUMMARY OF THE VACCINES MADE IN THE NETHERLANDS ON A
         ROUTINE BASIS

A. Human vaccines
- BCG: live bacterial vaccine
- Cholera: inactivated bacterial vaccine
- Diphtheria - tetanus - polio (DT-polio): mixed vaccine
- Diphtheria - pertussis - tetanus - polio (DPT-polio):
  polyvalent vaccine
- German measles (rubella): live viral vaccine
- Hepatitis B: inactivated viral vaccine
- Influenza: inactivated viral vaccine
- Measles: live viral vaccine
- Mumps: live viral vaccine
- Polio: inactivated viral vaccine
- Rabies: inactivated viral vaccine
- Tetanus: toxoid
- Typhoid: inactivated bacterial vaccine

B. Veterinary vaccines
   Poultry
- Avian encephalomyelitis: live viral vaccine
- Avian infectious bronchitis: live or inactivated viral
  vaccine, combined with others
- Avian infectious bursa disease (Gumboro disease): live or
  inactivated viral vaccine, combined with others
- Avian infectious laryngotracheitis: live viral vaccine

- Egg drop syndrome (EDS): inactivated viral vaccine, combined with others
- Fowl pox: live viral vaccine, combined with others
- Marek's disease: live viral vaccine
- Newcastle disease (NCD): inactivated or live viral vaccine, combined with others

Swine
- Atrophic rhinitis (Pasteurella multocida/Bordetella bronchiseptica): inactivated bacterial vaccine
- Pasteurella multocida: inactivated bacterial vaccine
- Aujeszky's disease: live or inactivated viral vaccine
- Clostridial infections: toxoid
- E. coli: inactivated bacterial vaccine
- Influenza: inactivated viral vaccine
- Erysipelas: inactivated bacterial vaccine

Cattle
- Brucella abortus: inactivated bacterial vaccine
- E. coli: inactivated bacterial vaccine
- Lungworm (husk): irradiated vaccine
- Anthrax: inactivated bacterial vaccine
- Foot-and-mouth disease: inactivated viral vaccine

Horse
- Influenza: inactivated viral vaccine
- Tetanus: toxoid

Dog
- Hepatitis: live or inactivated viral vaccine, combined with others
- Canine distemper: live or inactivated viral vaccine, combined with others
- Leptospirosis: live or inactivated bacterial vaccine, combined with others
- Measles: live viral vaccine
- Parvoviral infection: inactivated viral vaccine, combined with others
- Rabies: inactivated viral vaccine

Cat
- Herpesvirus, calicivirus and chlamydial infections: mixed live bacterial and viral vaccine

Canary
- Fowl pox: inactivated viral vaccine

Duck
- Hepatitis: live viral vaccine
- Fowl pest: live viral vaccine

Pigeon
- Fowl pox: live viral vaccine
- Salmonella typhimurium: inactivated bacterial vaccine
- Paramyxo-virus (PMV) disease: live or inactivated viral vaccine

Goose
- Hepatitis: live viral vaccine

28

4. QUALITY CONTROL

Although manufacturers strive for a consistent product by
choosing the appropriate starting material and standardization of
the production method, this cannot be guaranteed beforehand.
Numerous factors can influence the preparation of a vaccine
batch; for example, biological material is used and the
production process is complicated. As a result, one batch may
differ from another. Quality control of each separate batch is
consequently essential, both of the crude and of the purified
batch of toxoid or virus suspension during the production process
(the so-called in-process control) and of the end product during
the final stage (10, 11, 12).
Broadly, this quality control consists of two components, namely
(a) the safety test, and (b) the potency, or efficacy, test.
The classification given in Table 1 into bacterial, toxoid and
viral vaccines on the one hand, and live/attenuated and
inactivated vaccines on the other, is important for a review of
the types of tests involved in quality control. This is because
the type of agent and the nature of the vaccine product determine
how research and in particular _in vivo_ research will be
performed.

4.1. Safety evaluation
Testing the safety of the product is an integral part of the
batch control. This test ensures that the vaccine does not
contain ingredients harmful to man or animals after
administration. This harm can be traceable to:
a. the agent used (the bacterial strain, the toxin or the viral
   strain)
b. chemicals added to the vaccine product (intentionally or
   unintentionally)
c. the substrate used (culture medium, culture cells, embryonated
   hen's eggs, serum, vaccine liquid, etc.).

re a. Tests carried out as part of the safety control and which
      are aimed at possible harmful properties of the agent are:
      - the specific-toxicity test, to detect any residual
        virulence of live vaccine strains or incomplete
        inactivation of killed bacterial vaccines and toxoids. In
        the case of inactivated viral vaccines, the term virus
        inactivation test is used instead of specific-toxicity
        test. The specific-toxicity test is in many cases based
        on an _in vivo_ experiment;
      - the identity test, to ensure that the antigen in the
        vaccine is the same as that of the starting material. The
        reason is that, for example, containers of starting
        material may have been exchanged or packaging material
        incorrectly labelled.

re b. Various substances may be added to a vaccine during its
      production, such as adjuvants, preservatives, anti-foaming
      agents, inactivators, etc. The concentration of these
      substances is usually determined by chemical methods.
      Calamities may occur, for example, as a result of the use
      of chemically contaminated equipment. As regards the
      packaging process this can be checked by performing an
      abnormal-toxicity test on a number of ampoules containing
      the final product (called also innocuity test). Laboratory
      animals are used for this purpose.

For the veterinary vaccine control the abnormal-toxicity
test may be combined with the specific-toxicity test if the
examination is carried out on the target animal, and is
then referred to as the safety test.

re c. The substrate to be used in particular is a special risk
factor in the production of a vaccine. Animal components of
culture media as serum (for the bacterial vaccines and
toxoids) and culture cells, embryonated hen's eggs and
serum (for the viral vaccines) may be contaminated with
microorganisms or products thereof, especially when they
are derived from conventionally housed animals or animals
captured in the wild. In addition, there is the possibility
of contact-contamination of the substrate via the
personnel. Consequently, much attention is paid in the
safety examination to the detection of microbiological
contamination. There are several tests for this purpose:
- the sterility test. This is a general test for both
  bacterial and viral vaccines and its object is to detect
  contamination with bacteria, fungi and mycoplasmas. The
  sterility test is usually based on an _in vitro_ model.
- The test for extraneous microorganisms (that is,
  viruses). This test, which is restricted to the viral
  vaccines and the immunoglobulin preparations of animal
  origin, can be either an _in vitro_ or an _in vivo_ test
  (using cell cultures and embryonated eggs respectively).
- the test for the presence of endotoxins, that is,
  membrane components of Gram-negative bacteria. There is
  an _in vivo_ as well as _an vitro_ method for this.
  (Note: this test is not officially stipulated for the
  bacterial vaccines).

Since the introduction of subcultured cells (cells that have been
passaged more than once), continuous cell lines and cell strains
for virus production, these cells must not only be characterized
(identity, karyology) but also tested for possible malignant
properties. This so-called tumourigenicity test is performed _in
vivo_.
Table 2 gives a summary of the main safety tests for each vaccine
type.

4.2. Potency testing
A requisite for an effective vaccine is that it induces
protective immunity after its administration. Each batch should
be tested for this requirement. There is a large difference in
the design of the test between the live and the inactivated
vaccines. In the case of live, attenuated vaccine material (for
example, the BCG, rubella and the avian infectious bronchitis
vaccines), the efficacy of each vaccine batch is related to the
number of live particles, determined either by counting or by
titration, that is, entirely _in vitro_. Only when a new seed
strain is used is a once-only exhaustive potency test on animals
carried out. For veterinary vaccines, the seed-strain check
usually involves giving the target animal a lethal challenge
after immunization.
Unlike live vaccines, a potency test on each batch of inactivated
vaccine must be carried out, and this generally requires
experimental animals. The inactivated human influenza vaccine is
an exception, the determination of the vaccine's efficacy being
based on an _in vitro_ method, (single radial immunodiffusion).

Within the entire process of inactivated vaccine control,
relatively the most experimental animals are required for the
potency test.
Tables 3 and 4 give a summary of the control tests for a few
human bacterial vaccines and one viral vaccine, respectively,
during their successive production stages. They will be discussed
in the next chapter.

Table 2: SUMMARY OF SAFETY TESTS FOR BACTERIAL AND VIRAL VACCINES

<u>Bacterial vaccines</u>

<u>Live (attenuated)</u>   <u>Inactivated or toxoid</u>
 - Contaminating microorganisms*   - Sterility
 - Absence of virulent bacteria*   - Specific toxicity*
 - Identity*   - Identity*
 - Abnormal toxicity*   - Abnormal toxicity*

<u>Viral vaccines</u>

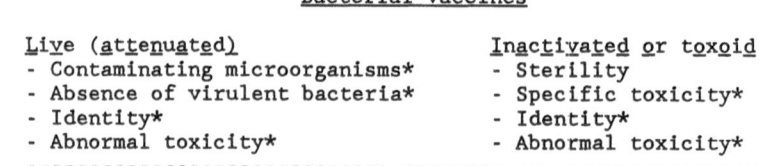

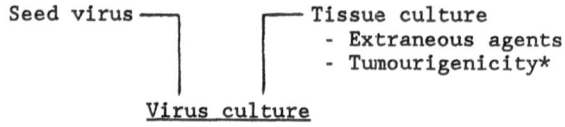

<u>Virus culture</u>

        <u>Live (attenuated)</u>   <u>Inactivated</u>
         - Sterility   - Sterility
         - Extraneous viruses*   - Extraneous viruses*
         - Specific toxicity*   - Inactivation*
         - Identity*   - Identity*
         - Abnormal toxicity*   - Abnormal toxicity*
----
* Requires animals
Note: This table gives a general outline. There may be subtle
      differences per vaccine product as regards test procedure.

Table 3: CONTROL TESTS OF A FEW HUMAN BACTERIAL VACCINES DURING
          THEIR SUCCESSIVE PRODUCTION STAGES (13)

     Diphtheria and tetanus   Pertussis

```
     ┌──────────┐   - -"crude bulk" - -   ┌──────────┐
     │  toxin   │                         │ bacterial│
     │ harvest  │                         │ harvest  │
     └──────────┘                         └──────────┘
         │ -sterility test                    │ -sterility test
         │ -antigenicity determination        │ -potency test*
         │  (=the Lf test)
     ┌──────────┐
     │  Crude   │
     │ toxoid   │
     └──────────┘
         │ -sterility test
         │ -specific-toxicity test*
         │ -Lf test
     ┌──────────┐   -"purified bulk"-     ┌──────────┐
     │ Purified │                         │ initial  │
     │ toxoid   │                         │ bulk     │
     └──────────┘                         └──────────┘
         │ -sterility test                    │ -sterility test
         │ -specific-toxicity test*           │ -specific
         │                                    │  toxicity test*
         │ -chemical assays                   │ -potency test*
         │                ┌──────────┐        │
         └────────────────│  Final   │────────┘
                          │  bulk    │
                          └──────────┘
                               │ -sterility test
                               │ -specific-toxicity test*
                               │ -potency test*
                               │ -chemical assays
                          ┌──────────┐
                          │ Final lot│
                          └──────────┘
                               │ -chemical assays
                               │ -sterility test
                               │ -identity test*
                               │ -abnormal-toxicity test*
```

* Requires test animals

Table 4: CONTROL TESTS ON THE RABIES VACCINE DURING ITS
         SUCCESSIVE PRODUCTION STAGES (14)

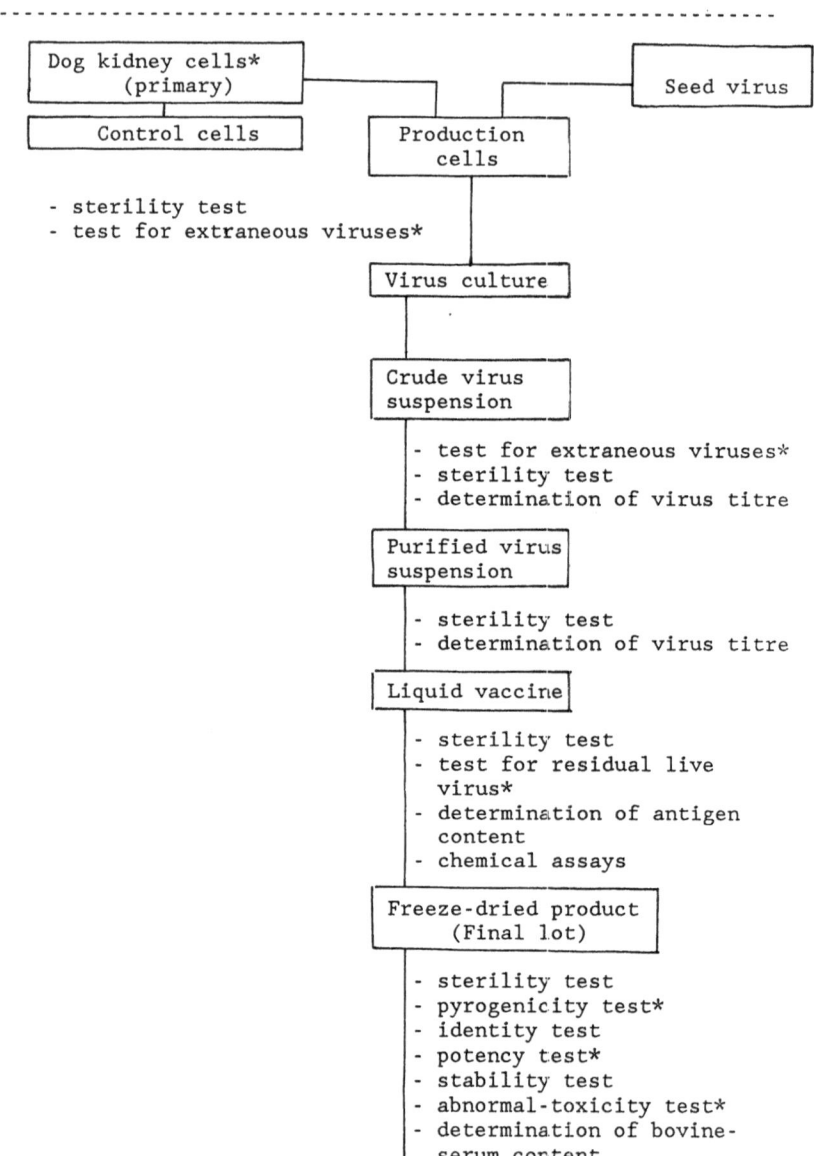

* Requires test animals

5. GUIDELINES

In many countries the production and quality control of human and
veterinary vaccines are regulated by Acts. In the Netherlands
this has been the case for the human vaccines since 1927 and for
the veterinary vaccines from 1986. In most countries compliance
with these Acts is supervised by a special committee which
delegates the actual work to the National Control Laboratory
(NCL). This laboratory is generally authorized to inspect
production centres throughout the country, to re-test vaccines
produced at home and abroad, and to develop and adapt guidelines.
All vaccines have to be approved by the NCL before they can be
released for general use. However, the manufacturer remains at
all times responsible for its own products.
Manufacturers use their own specifications for vaccine production
and quality control. These are generally based on the official
guidelines of the country of production or those of the importing
country. In addition, the guidelines of the WHO and of the
European Pharmacopoeia are relevant because of their
supranational and international status; those of the WHO for
human products and those of the European Pharmacopoeia for both
human and veterinary vaccines.
For this reason, a brief note on both the WHO and the European
Pharmacopoeia are here considered relevant.
The WHO has long been striving for international standardization
of the quality of biological products. In the first instance it
distributed only standard preparations for the calibration of
national reference preparations, but since the sixties it has
also been increasingly involved in drawing up guidelines for
quality control. For this purpose, there is a special WHO
committee, the "Expert Committee on Biological Standardization",
which can appoint ad hoc Working Parties to address specific
issues. Guidelines are published in the Technical Report Series
and are intended as recommendations. It is left to the national
control authorities to decide whether to incorporate these into
the law of the individual countries.
The establishment of the European Pharmacopoeia is the outcome of
the Convention on the Elaboration of a European Pharmacopoeia,
under the auspices of the Council of Europe. Its first meeting
took place in July 1964. Meanwhile, 17 West-European countries
have joined this Convention. Under articles 3 to 6 inclusive of
this Convention, two bodies of the Council of Europe are
responsible for implementing the European Pharmacopoeia, namely:
-    the Public Health Committee, composed of official
     representatives of the Ministries of Health of the
     participating countries. This Committee has a policy-making
     function.
-    the European Pharmacopoeia Commission, a technical and
     scientific body comprising experts from the participating
     countries, which is concerned with the content of the
     guidelines.
The guidelines are published in the form of monographs. Each
monograph covers the specifications for one medical product as
regards its quality control. Up to 1987, monographs on 40
different human and veterinary vaccine products had appeared
(Table 5), and monographs on other products are in preparation.

34

Table 5: THE EDITIONS OF THE EUROPEAN PHARMACOPOEIA. THE NUMBER
OF MONOGRAPHS ON VACCINES AND THE TOTAL NUMBER OF
ANIMAL TESTS PRESCRIBED IN THE MONOGRAPHS

	Number of vaccine monographs	Total number of animal experiments
1st Edition, vol.2 (1971)	14	24
1st Edition, vol.3 Suppl. (1977)	11	43
2nd Edition, (from 1980)	26	72

The guidelines formulated in the monographs must be implemented by the countries wich have signed the Convention, unless stated otherwise in the monograph (15).

International harmonization of guidelines and regulations and a mutual recognition of the results of animal tests by different countries are in the interest of animal reduction and refinement and will therefore be discussed later (chapter 12, section 2).

6. GOOD MANUFACTURING PRACTICE (GMP)

The development, production and testing of vaccines should be specified in such a way that the quality of the product is adequately assured. In the past few years, in particular, the emphasis has been on this quality control and the concept of Good Manufacturing Practice (GMP) has found general acceptance. In short, GMP embodies the complete set of guidelines relating to the quality of the product and the monitoring of that quality. These guidelines concern, among other things, the qualifications of the relevant personnel, hygiene, documentation and responsibilities. In a positive sense, GMP can help to reduce the use of experimental animals, because improvement of both the product and its control decreases the need for re-testing, for example, by the NCL.

7. REFERENCES

1. Dekking, F. et al.: Immunisatie tegen infectieziekten (Immunization against infectious diseases), Vol. 89 in the series entitled Nederlandse Bibliotheek der Geneeskunde (Dutch Medical Library), 1974, published by Stafleu's Wetenschappelijke Uitgeversmaatschappij B.V., Leiden.
2. Dudgeon, J.A.: Immunization in times ancient and modern. Journ. Roy. Soc. Med. (1980), 73, 581-586.
3. Dudgeon, J.A.: The control of diphtheria, tetanus, poliomyelitis, measles, rubella and mumps. Practitioner, (1975), 215 (1287), 299-309.
4. McIntyre, L.: The malaria vaccine. Publ. Hlth. Lond. (1985), 99, 343-348.
5. Grzych, J.M. et al.: An anti-idiotype vaccine against experimental schistosomiasis. Nature (1985), vol. 316, 74.
6. Enders, J.F. et al.: Cultivation of the Lansing strain of poliomyelitis virus in cultures of various human embryonic tissues. Science, (1949), 247, 12, 1726-1728.
7. Ruitenberg, E.J.: Vaccinbereiding (Preparation of Vaccines). Natuur en Techniek, (1984), 52, 11, 978-991.
8. Berlin, B.S. et al.: Rhesus diploid rabies vaccine (adsorbed), a new rabies vaccine. JAMA, (1982), 247, 12, 1726-1728.
9. Wezel, A.L. van, et al.: New approach to the production of concentrated and purified inactivated polio and rabies tissue culture vaccines. Develop. Biol. Standard. (1978), 41, 159-168.
10. Perkins, F.T.: Safety of vaccines. Brit. Med. Bull. (1969), 25, 208-212.
11. Perkins, F.T.: Safety testing of vaccines. Symp. Series immunobiol. Standard. (1973), 22, 177-182.
12. Starke, G. and Hlinak, P.: Requirements for the control of a dog kidney cell adapted live mumps virus vaccine. Journ. Biol. Standard. (1974), 2, 143-150.
13. Dutch National Institute of Public Health and Environmental Protection (RIVM): Vaccine control course, Course Book (1984).
14. Steenis, G. van et al.: Nederlands celkweek-rabiesvaccin voor toepassing bij de mens. (Dutch cell-cultured rabies vaccine for human use.) Ned. Tijdschr. Geneeskd. (1984), 128, 38, 1810-1814.
15. The European Pharmacopoeia: A review of its history and functions, Maisonneuve, 1981.

CHAPTER 5: EXPERIMENTAL ANIMALS AND ANIMAL EXPERIMENTS

In the last chapter the importance of animal experimentation for the current production and control of vaccines has already been referred to several times without discussing its substance. This subject will be elaborated in the following sections with special attention devoted to the extent, purpose and relevance of this research and the pain or distress suffered by laboratory animals.

1. EXTENT OF THE RESEARCH

From a historical viewpoint, there exists a close and long-standing association between laboratory animal and vaccine, although it is difficult to substantiate this statement by figures. In Britain, Statistics of Experiments on Living Animals (1) have been published annually since 1876 when the Cruelty to Animals Act* came into force. It has long been the only country with a detailed survey of laboratory animal use.
However, data on the extent and purpose of the use of animals are now available for other countries, for example, Norway, Danmark, Switzerland and the Netherlands. In the Netherlands, this information is provided by the establishments where laboratory animals are used since 1977, when the Animal Experimentation Act became law. This Act also introduced the annual registration and publication of information concerning, among other things, the numbers of laboratory animals used by licence-holders (mandatory since 1986). The data collected reveal that 1,208,539 animals were used by the biomedical sciences in 1986, representing a reduction of 24 per cent over the 1978 figure, the first year of registration. Apart from Britain, where 3.1 million animals were used in 1986 (1), Norway: 111.600 and Switzerland: 1.4 million few accurate figures are available for other countries. Estimates of the number of animals used every year are 1 million in India, 6 million in Japan, 2 million in Canada and 17-20 million in the United States (2). The number of animals used worldwide is estimated at 100 (3) to 200 (4) million annually. It is also difficult to indicate what proportion of the animals was used for vaccine purposes, even for those countries with detailed statistics. Question 1 on the Dutch registration forms concerns the purpose of the experiment (figure 1). One of the categories is the production, testing or biological standardization of sera, vaccines and other biological products, such as blood products, insulin and monoclonal antibodies. However, the registration does not allow this category to be further specified, but it may assumed that vaccine research is the major user of animals. On the basis of data from table 1 the number of animals used annually for this purpose would be at least 50%, or 125,000, corresponding to about 10% of the total number of animals used. This percentage is in broad agreement with the situation in Britain (5). If the 10% percentage was applicable worldwide then the total figure would be in the range of 10 to 20 million animals used every year.

---

* The 1876 Act was repeated on 1 January 1987 and replaced by the Animals (Scientific Procedures) Act 1986.

38

Figure 1. TOTAL NUMBER OF ANIMALS USED IN THE NETHERLANDS IN
1986: 1,208,539.

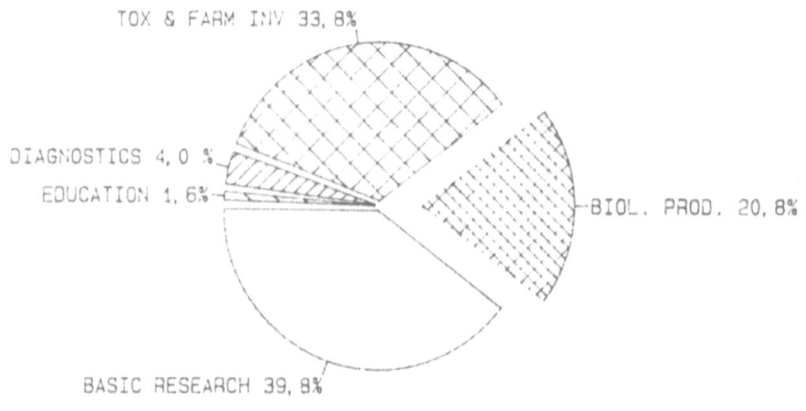

Table 1: NUMBERS OF ANIMALS USED IN THE CATEGORY OF BIOLOCAL
PRODUCTS IN THE NETHERLANDS, 1980-1986 (6)

Year	No. of animals	% of total
1980	234,490	15.77
1981	288,400	19.92
1982	267,900	18.84
1983	266,800	20.07
1984	230,000	18.53
1985	226,830	19.30
1986	250,950	20.80

Since detailed and accurate figures are available on the usage of
animals in the production and quality control of biological
products in the Netherlands, they are here discussed briefly as
an example. For each species, the total number of animals used
and the numbers used for biological products are given in table
2. One striking feature is the relatively high percentage of
mice, guinea pigs, rabbits and birds (chiefly poultry) and the
relatively low percentage of rats.

Table 2: ANIMAL SPECIES, AND FOR EACH SPECIES THE TOTAL NUMBER
USED AND THE PERCENTAGE OF THE TOTAL IN THE CATEGORY OF
BIOLOGICAL PRODUCTS IN THE NETHERLANDS IN 1986 (6).

Animal species	Total no. of experimental animals	No. used for biological products	Percentage of the total
Total	1,208,539	250,950	20.8
Mouse	595,412	165,086	27.7
Rat	341,771	11,783	3.4
Guinea pig	27,134	10,265	37.8
Other rodents	11,020	1,825	16.6
Rabbit	16,892	7,602	45.0
Monkey	553	93	16.8
Dog	2,743	331	12.1
Cat	1,036	74	7.1
Other carnivores	175	14	8.0
Horse	182	10	5.5
Swine	9,105	1,613	17.7
Sheep and goat	1,958	323	16.5
Ruminants	2,053	298	14.5
Other mammels	31	15	48.4
Birds	99,687	51,367	51.5
Amphibia	1,468	53	3.6
Fish	97,161	202	0.2

Some other features of research on experimental animals for
vaccine control can be deduced from annual registration forms
returned by licence-holder. For example, in 1986, the answers to
the following questions were:
- Was the experiment directly or indirectly of importance to the
  health and feeding of man or animals?

Biological products		Total	
Yes:	100%	Yes:	98%
No:	0%	No:	2%

- Was the experiment performed in order to comply with statutory
  regulations?

Biological products		Total	
Yes:	55%	Yes:	29%
No:	45%	No:	71%

This response is related to the purpose of animal tests for
vaccines, which can be characterized in particular by such key
words as "applied", "routine", and "quality controlling".
In addition, some animals are used in this field for improving
the existing animal tests and developing new ones.

2. PURPOSE OF THE RESEARCH

The human and veterinary vaccines produced in the Netherlands
were surveyed in Chapter 4. Any classification of the number of
animals required annually for each vaccine product would only
have limited value because this number depends on the production
volume (number of batches) and this may vary from year to year.
Table 3, which gives figures for the human bacterial vaccines,
should therefore be interpreted with some caution.

Table 3: NUMBER OF EXPERIMENTAL ANIMALS USED IN THE NETHERLANDS
         IN 1983 AND 1986 FOR HUMAN BACTERIAL VACCINES (7)

Vaccine	No. of animals used in 1983	No. of animals used in 1986
BCG	580	126
Cholera	800	181
Diphtheria	7,600	4,171
Pertussis	19,000	21,156
Meningococci (experimental)	2,300	1,848
Tetanus	7,600	3,800
Typhoid	550	6

However, it is possible to classify the various vaccine products
according to the number of animals used for both in-process and
final control of each vaccine batch (see table 4). The number of
animals given in this table is in accordance with the Dutch
regulations.
It can be deduced from this survey that in general the total
number of animals required for the bacterial vaccines is greater
than that for the viral vaccines, and that it is greater for the
inactivated (human) vaccines than for the live products. To
obtain further information about the purpose for which the
animals are used a distinction should be made between production
and quality control.

Table 4: SUMMARY OF THE NUMBER OF ANIMALS REQUIRED FOR THE
TESTING OF ONE VACCINE BATCH

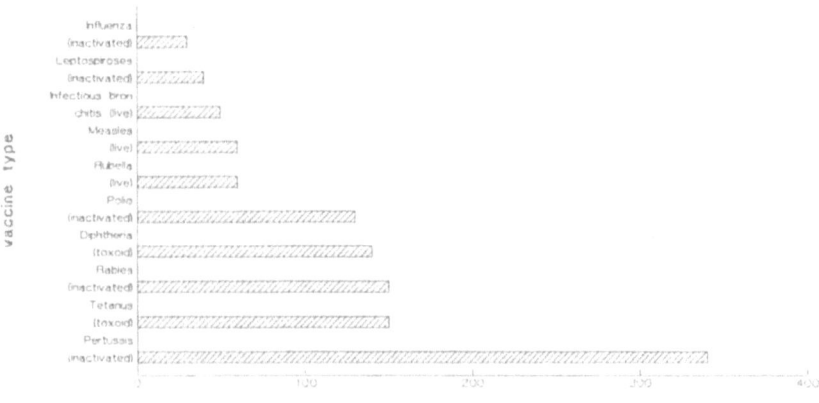

No. of animals / batch

2.1. production

The animal plays only a minor role in the preparation of
bacterial vaccines. Only for the culture media are animal
products such as serum or blood sometimes required. The situation
is somewhat different as regards the viral vaccines. In a few
countries, some vaccine viruses such as, for example, rabies, are
still propagated in vivo. Most Western countries, however, use
only embryonated (hen) eggs or cell cultures (see table 5). These
cells are derived directly from animals where primary cultures
are used, and animals are sacrificed for this purpose. The pain
and distress involved here falls in the category "slight"
according to the rating of the experimental animal registration.
The number of animals needed for vaccine production is being
gradually reduced through the replacement of primary cultures by
subcultured cells (tertiary cells for polio). Thus, at present,
the production of (inactivated) polio vaccine in the Netherlands
requires about 30 monkeys and that of rabies vaccine only one dog
(8).

Table 5: ORIGIN OF THE CELL CULTURES USED FOR THE PRODUCTION OF
VIRAL VACCINES

Poliomyelitis (inact.)	Rabies (inact.)	Measles (live,atten.)	Rubella (live,atten.)
monkey	dog	chicken	rabbit
	chicken	dog	dog
	rabbit	guinea pig	duck
	human diploid cells	monkey (Vero cell line)	guinea pig
			human diploid cells

2.2. Quality control

The importance of quality control was pointed out in chapter 4.
Tables 3 and 4 in that chapter showed that there are various
animal tests available for this purpose. Most of them can,
however, be reduced to a limited number of basic principles and
techniques, mainly relating to the testing for safety and
efficacy of the product.
Table 6 summarizes the various animal tests involved; they are
described below. It should be realised that only a general
description is given, and that the test procedure may vary
according to the particular vaccine or vaccine type being
examined.

Table 6: TESTS PERFORMED IN EXPERIMENTAL ANIMALS FOR
         QUALITYCONTROL

Safety evaluation: - Test for specific toxicity
                   - Test for freedom from extraneous
                       microorganisms
                   - Test for residual live virus
                   - Tumourigenicity test
                   - Safety test
                   - Identity test
                   - Test for abnormal toxicity

Potency testing : - Qualitative assays
                   - Quantitative assays

2.2.1. Safety evaluation

- Test for specific toxicity
  The purpose of this test is to detect any incomplete
  inactivation of the vaccine product. It is an integral part of
  the quality control (both in-process and final testing) of the
  inactivated human bacterial vaccines. Groups of animals (guinea
  pigs for diphtheria and tetanus; mice for pertussis) are
  injected with a dose of the crude or purified product several
  times greater than that used to immunize humans.
  For the toxoid vaccines, the criterion is the occurrence of
  clinical symptoms or of macroscopic changes. The safety test
  for pertussis vaccine is based on the effect of incompletely
  inactivated pertussis bacteria on the weight gain of mice.

- Test for freedom from extraneous microorganisms
  Animal tissues, embryonated eggs and sera which are used for
  the production of the viral vaccines may be a potential source
  of extraneous microorganisms (in particular viruses), even -
  albeit to a much lesser extent - when they are derived from
  specific-pathogen-free (SPF) animals. In addition,
  contamination may occur through contact with personnel or the
  equipment employed. Hence, testing for extraneous
  microorganisms is an important part of the quality control of
  virus vaccines.
  Many, but not all, extraneous viruses (for example, the
  lymphocytic choriomeningitis (LCM) virus) can be detected by in
  vitro methods (cell cultures). Testing for extraneous
  microorganisms therefore consists of performing various
  complementary tests, including one or more involving animals.

For the human viral vaccines, intraperitoneal and intracerebral administration of the vaccine to adult or newborn mice is a standard procedure. Apart from mice, other animal species such as the rabbit, dog or guinea pig can also be used for this. Assessment criteria are the occurrence of clinical symptoms and/or macroscopic changes and/or specific antibodies in the blood serum. There are three complementary tests for live poultry vaccines, namely, one performed in cell cultures, one in embryonated hen's eggs and one in chicks. In the case of the other veterinary vaccines, a specific animal model is not required for testing for extraneous microorganisms. This examination is usually part of a combined test.

- Test for residual live virus
Vaccines prepared from inactivated virus strains must be examined during the production process for the presence of non-inactivated vaccine virus. In many cases this can be done in cell cultures. For the rabies vaccine there is also an animal test in which the virus suspension is administered intracerebrally to a group of mice. The presence of rabies virus causes clinical symptoms or death. The test in monkeys for residual live virus in the (inactivated) polio vaccine has recently been discontinued in most countries, except the U.S.A.

- Tumourigenicity test
Cells used for the production of virus vaccines and not derived from primary cultures may possess oncogenic properties. These cells are not accepted for the production of human vaccines. Part of the current requirements concerning the acceptability of subcultured cells or cell lines is therefore the absence of tumourigenic properties. This can be tested by means of various animal models, all involving immunosuppressed animals. Various models exist for tumourigenicity testing. As a rule, 2 groups of animals are used (immunosuppressed rats, mice or hamsters). One of the groups serves as a control and is injected subcutaneously with specific tumour cells, while the other group is given a subcutaneous injection of cells from the production culture. The criterion is the development of tumours at the site of injection (and - in some guidelines -metastases).

- Safety test
In the control of vaccines for veterinary use, the test for possible harmfulness can be performed in the target animal. This enables several safety tests to be combined, such as the tests for abnormal and specific toxicity, for residual live virus and for extraneous microorganisms.
The testing procedure for most vaccines for use in mammals consists of administering a multiple dose of the product to 2 animals of the species for which it is intended. With poultry vaccines, larger groups of animals (10-25) are normally used and the dose is different for each vaccine product. The commonly used criterion is the development of symptoms during the observation period.

- Identity test
The identity of a product can often be established by an in vitro technique. One example is the demonstration of the presence tetanus toxin or toxoid with the help of specific antibodies in the Lf assay.

44

When the identity test is based on an _in vivo_ technique, it consists of demonstrating specific antibodies in the animal after immunization, either by challenging with the (virulent) microorganism (or toxin) or by a serum-antibody assay.

- Test for abnormal toxicity
  The aim of this test is to detect any unknown contamination of the vaccine and it is performed on the final lot. The testing procedure is simple and identical for nearly all vaccine types. Each of 2 guinea pigs receives 5 human doses and each of 2-5 mice one human dose of the vaccine. The animals should remain healthy and show no weight loss.
  In the case of the veterinary vaccines, this test can be combined with another one if the target species is used (9).

2.2.2. Potency testing

For background information about the purpose of this examination the reader is referred to chapter 4. As regards the effectiveness of a vaccine, a distinction was made in this chapter between the determination of the amount of antigen (referred to as antigenicity assay) and the determination of the capacity to induce protective immunity (the immunogenicity assay).
In the case of live vaccines, the antigenicity assay, which is an _in vitro_ assay based on counting or culturing the vaccine microorganism, is sufficient for batch testing. This is partly because replication of vaccine virus or bacterium still continues in the vaccinee's body after administration. The inactivated vaccines lack this capacity and only the amount of antigen present in the vaccine liquid contributes to building up immunity.
Although there is strictly speaking a correlation between the amount of antigen and the protective immunity induced by it, this correlation is not constant. Various factors can affect the potency of the antigen, such as the mode and site of administration, or the addition of an adjuvant, mixing with other products (the pertussis vaccine, for example, potentiates the immune response to the tetanus vaccine, table 7).

Table 7. EFFECT OF THE PERTUSSIS COMPONENT ON THE EFFICACY OF THE TETANUS VACCINE IN A MULTIVALENT PRODUCT (11)

Composition	DT-polio	DPT-polio
D (diphtheria)	2.5 Lf/ml	15 Lf/ml
T (tetanus)	5 Lf/ml	5 Lf/ml
P (pertussis)	---	10 IOU
AlPO$_4$	1.5 Lf/ml	1.5 mg/ml
Efficacy of tetanus component	71 ± 10 IU/ml	171 ± 43 IU/ml

Lf = Limes flocculation; IOU = International Opacity Units;
IU = International Units; AlPO$_4$ is used as an adjuvant.
Note: it is known that the diphtheria component does not affect the efficacy of the tetanus component.

For these reasons, the use of in vitro antigenicity assays, such as the Lf method for tetanus and diphtheria and the ELISA for polio, is restricted to in-process control of vaccine products. An immunogenicity assay is essential for the quality control of the final product and these assays are nearly always based on animal models. The animal species used is usually not the same as the target species, and with the human vaccines it is never the same. This means that most immunogenicity assays are artificial as regards design and performance. There are differences, for example, regarding the mode of administration, the dose, the frequency of administration and the determination of the end-point. The immunogenicity test can be carried out in one of two ways. In one a (small) group of animals is immunized with the vaccine, followed by a challenging dose of the virulent microorganism in question. In the other the vaccine is injected into the animals, samples of blood are taken and the specific antibody titre measured*.

The criterion for this qualitative assay is based on the "pass or fail" principle, the relevant vaccine being passed if a given number of animals survives the challenge or shows no clinical symptoms, or if the mean serum antibody titre exceeds a given lower limit.

The value of the qualitative assay methods is limited by the fact that the outcome is influenced by the experimental conditions (see chapter 3).

This applies to a lesser extent to quantitative assay methods, where a relationship is established statistically between vaccine dose and potency of the product. The principle of the quantitative assay consists of administering different vaccine dilutions to groups of experimental animals. In the case of veterinary vaccines, a control group is usually included. For the human vaccines, a reference vaccine of known immunogenicity is normally used. Groups of animals are injected with dilutions of the reference preparation parallel to the vaccine under examination. The protective immunity is measured after an immunization period, which is dependent on the vaccine used. In a few cases it is sufficient to take a blood sample and determine the antibody titre in the blood serum. With most products, however, the animals are challenged with the virulent microorganism or toxin. The vaccine dilutions are usually so chosen that there is a high mortality rate with the highest vaccine dilution and a high survival rate whith the lowest vaccine dilution. Alternatives to the death criterion to measure the potency of a vaccine are paralysis (paralytic challenge), skin reaction (dermal challenge) and clinical symptoms (clinical challenge). On the basis of the criteria used, the ED50 (see chapter 4 for a definition) or the PI50** of the vaccine under examination can be analyzed statistically, and in the case of ____

---

* In general, the amount of antibodies is measured by in vitro methods such as an ELISA or haemagglutination. Since the antibody content measured by these methods need not a priori correspond to the content of neutralizing (protective) antibodies, the introduction of these techniques must be preceded by thorough validation.

** A variant of the ED50 which is applied to several veterinary vaccines (e.g. E.coli) is based on one vaccine dilution and graded challenging doses. Statistical analysis of the data obtained gives the Protective Index 50 or PI50.

human vaccines, also the potency of the product in relation to the reference preparation. The types of potency assay used are given in table 8 for each vaccine product.

Table 8: POTENCY TESTS ON INACTIVATED HUMAN AND VETERINARY VACCINES

Vaccine	in vitro	quantitative challenge				quantitative serology	qualitative challenge	qualitative serology	use of reference preparation
		L	D	P	C				
Cholera		X						X	X
Diphtheria (human)		X	X						X
Influenza (human)	X								
Pertussis		X							X
Poliomyelitis				X					X
Rabies (human)		X							X
Tetanus		X	X						X
Typhoid							X	X	
*Infect. bronchitis								X	
*Egg drop syndrome					X				
*Newcastle disease		X					X		
Atropic rhinitis		X							
*Aujeszky's disease		X							
Clostridium		X							
*E. coli (swine)		X							
*Influenza (swine)					X				
*Brucella abortus				X					
*E. coli (cattle)		X							
Anthrax		X							
Foot-and-mouth dis.				X					
Influenza (equine)								X	
*Hepatitis (canine)								X	
*Canine distemper								X	
Leptospirosis		X							
*Parvoviral infection								X	
*Rabies (veterinary)		X							X
*Gumboro disease					X				

L - lethal challenge   D - dermal challenge
P - paralytic challenge   C - clinical challenge
* - tested in accordance with the Dutch specifications

3. RELEVANCE OF THE TESTS

In recent years there has been a rapid development of in vitro techniques for application in the quality control of vaccine products. Nevertheless, the experimental animal is still the main indicator in the detection of desirable or undesirable activities of newly produced vaccine batches. In general, this activity is well-defined and the animal test has a specific purpose, for example, that of determining the effectiveness or the specific toxicity of the product. Occasionally the test is of a general empirical nature and its purpose is not so clear-cut. This is especially true of the test for abnormal toxicity, which is aimed at detecting any unknown contamination of the final product. For the human vaccines, in particular, where fundamental research on the "target animal" - man - is for obvious reasons almost impossible, the development of a good animal model requires considerable effort. Moreover, an assessment of the relevance of the model can only be made after validating it by comparison with human data.

These data are generally based on the outcome of field trials in which the vaccine is administered to a sufficiently large population under controlled conditions. Data resulting from these trials can be of retrospective value for adapting and improving the animal model and thus for the relevance of the model. It is therefore advisable to conduct field trials. However, such a trial is difficult, expensive and not always practicable. For this reason it is sometimes uncertain whether the animal model employed in a routine manner has sufficient predictive value. This applies, for example, to the current animal tests to estimate the potency of the cholera vaccine (12). On the other hand, in several other cases this correlation between animal model and man has been established. Examples include the animal potency tests of the tetanus (13) and the pertussis (14, 15) vaccines, the specific toxicity test on the latter (16), and recently the quality control tests on the purified (Sato) pertussis vaccine.

4. DISTRESS

The annual survey of the usage of experimental animals in the Netherlands includes a question about the degree of distress suffered by the animals as a result of the experimental procedure. Distress is here defined as a condition in which the animal's health is impaired, or as considerable pain, injury or other severe distress inflicted on the animal (17). The registration booklet "Records of experimental animals and animal tests" which is sent every year to the licence holders by the Veterinary Chief Inspectorate for Public Health, distinguishes 6 degrees of distress:

1 - slight
2 - moderate
3 - severe, lasting less than one day
4 - severe, lasting 1-7 days
5 - severe, lasting 7-30 days
6 - severe, lasting more than 30 days

Table 9 gives a list of the various degrees of distress inflicted on animals in the quality control of biological products. It shows that the distress caused here is more severe than for other kinds of biomedical research. As part of the present project, a specification of this distress was made for the quality-control tests. To this end, the relevant data on a number of vaccine products were collected. One notable feature, not entirely unexpected, was the finding that a particular technique was not rated uniformly. Distress or pain is a subjective concept which means different things to different people. Criteria for each degree of distress cannot be defined in such a way as to leave no room for a variety of views. Furthermore, the degree of distress need not be the same for each animal within one test. An example is the potency test which involves a control group as well as a test group. Control animals receive no vaccine and are thus not protected against a challenge, whereas the immunized animals are usually protected depending on the vaccine dose given.

Table 9: NUMBERS OF EXPERIMENTAL ANIMALS USED IN 1986 IN THE
NETHERLANDS FOR THE PRODUCTION, TESTING AND BIOLOGICAL
STANDARDIZATION OF BIOLOGICALS, CATAGORISED BY DISTRESS
RATING (1)

Distress	All fields		Biological products	
	number	%	number	%
slight	646,524	53,5	96,187	38,3
moderate	274,343	22,7	61,177	24,4
severe (<1 day)	79,086	6,5	5,507	2,2
severe (1-7 days)	165,996	13,7	76,594	30,5
severe (7-30 days)	38,343	3,2	11,421	4,6
severe (>30 days)	4,247	0,3	68	0,03

When assessing the amount of suffering inflicted, some
manufacturers start from the suffering that may arise and assign
all the animals to category 4 while others distinguish between
the control group (category 4) and the immunized group (category
1). A guideline for dealing with such cases could eliminate this
discrepancy. An additional recommendation for internal use within
an institute could be to make a double assessment of the degree
of distress inflicted, the first one being of the anticipated
suffering at the beginning of the experiment, the second of the
actual distress at the end of the test. This would make it
possible for both the experimenter and the animal expert
responsable to recognize immediately the abnormal course of any
experiment.
For the animal tests performed as part of the human vaccine
control, the numbers of animals to be used and the degree of
distress (distress rating) are summarized in table 10. It shows
clearly that particular attention should be paid to the potency
assay when aiming at reduction or refinement in the utilisation
of laboratory animals.

Table 10: THE NUMBERS OF ANIMALS REQUIRED AND DISTRESS RATING FOR
THE VARIOUS TESTS USED IN THE QUALITY CONTROL OF EACH
BATCH OF HUMAN VACCINE

Animal test	Approx. no. of animals	distress rating
Potency	100	severe (4)
Tumourigenicity	20	severe (4)
Specific toxicity	20-80	slight to severe (4)
Freedom from extraneous microorganisms	30	slight (1)
Abnormal toxicity	7	slight (1)

Note: the data on the potency test are based on the lethal
challenge procedure.

5. REFERENCES

1. Home Office (1987). Statistics of Experiments on Living Animals in Great Britain 1986 (Cm 187). London: Home Office.
2. OTA (Office of Technology Assessment) Alternatives to animal use in research, testing and education. The Johns Hopkins Center for Alternatives to Animal Testing. Newsletter (1985), 2, 3-4.
3. Hampson, J.E. and Silcock, S.R.: 9th European public parliamentary hearing on the use of live animals for experimental and industrial purposes (1982), 34, 5.
4. Howard-Jones, N.: A CIOMS ethical code for animal experimentation. WHO Chronicle, (1985), 39, 2, 51-56.
5. Silcock, S.R.: Personal communication.
6. Zo doende (Animal experimentation in the Netherlands, Statistics) 1981, 1982, 1983, 1984, 1985, 1986. Veterinary Chief Inspectorate for Public Health, Animal Experiments Department, Rijswijk, the Netherlands.
7. de Graaf, W.F.J. and Kreeftenberg, J.C.: Department of Animal Experimentation, Laboratory for Control of Bacterial Vaccines, 1983 and 1986. Report of the National Institute of Public Health and Environmental Hygiene (RIVM).
8. Kruijt, B.C.: Personal communication.
9. European Pharmacopoeia, 2nd Edition (1980), 62, vaccina ad usum veterinarium.
10. Sheffield, F.: Use of animals in the quality control of vaccines. Journ. Roy. Soc. Med. (1978), 71, 677-682.
11. Kreeftenberg, J.C. et al.: A mouse model to estimate the potency of the diphtheria component in combined vaccines. Develop. Biol. Standard. (1986), 64, 21-24.
12. Sinha, V.B. and Bhaskaran, K.: Immunity in experimental cholera: effect of parenteral immunization with vaccines and toxoid. Bull. Wld. Hlth. Org. (1973), 49, 605-613.
13. Ramshorst, J.D. van et al.: The relation between animal potency tests and the human response to adsorbed tetanus toxoids. Journ. Biol. Standard. (1973), 1, 215-220.
14. Standfast, A.F.B.: The comparison between field trials and mouse protection tests against intranasal and intracerebral challenges with Bordetella pertussis. Immunology, (1958), 2, 135-143.
15. Medical Research Council: Vaccination against whooping-cough: relation between protection in children and results of laboratory tests. Brit. Med. J. (1956), 2, 454.
16. Pittman, M. and Cox, C.B.: Pertussis vaccine testing for freedom-from-toxicity. Applied Microbiol. (1965), 13, 3, 447-456.
17. Records of experimental animals and animal tests. Veterinary Chief Inspectorate for Public Health, Animal Experiments Department, Rijswijk, the Netherlands

CHAPTER 6: ANIMAL EXPERIMENTATION AND ITS SHORTCOMINGS

Despite the fact that animal experiments are performed on a large
scale and their value for biomedical research is beyond doubt,
the use of animals for this purpose is increasingly being
criticized not only by the general public but also by the
scientific community. The importance and value of animal
experimentation have been discussed in the previous chapters. The
limitations of this type of research will now be considered.

1. INTRODUCTION

On the basis of existing knowledge, there is a concensus within
-and also mostly outside - the scientific establishment on the
need for animal experiments to maintain and promote the welfare
of the community. It is precisely for this reason that the
improvement of the animal model should be given priority. It is
obvious that breeding animals specifically for research and
keeping them in the best possible health by providing good
housing and environmental conditions, proper diet and care will
make a positive contribution to the value of research. In many
cases this makes it possible to reduce the number of animals
required. Good animal husbandry is therefore just as much a form
of animal protection as are the socially or politically accepted
ways. Nevertheless, the scientifically justifiable use of animals
in experiments should not be regarded as the definitive solution
to the issue of animal experimentation. This is because animal
experimentation involves aspects which argue for making
biomedical research in general and vaccine research in particular
less dependent on the laboratory animal. These aspects are here
briefly discussed.

2. LIMITATIONS OF ANIMAL EXPERIMENTATION

2.1. Moral aspects
In recent years there has been a change in the way people think
about animals. A better understanding of the animal, particularly
in the physiological and ethological fields, have led us to
question whether it is right to treat animals as mere objects
serving our needs and wishes, and the growing interest in the
issues raised by animal experimentation can be explained in that
light.
Until recently, laboratory animals were considered to be of
instrumental value only. However, it is increasingly being
recognized that animals also have an intrinsic value, and that
they have a life of their own. For example, the "Proposed
International Guiding Principles for Biomedical Research
Involving Animals" of the CIOMS (The Council for International
Organizations of Medical Sciences) (1) and the Memorandum
"Experimental animal policy" of the Dutch Ministry of Welfare,
Public Health and Culture (2) use the term "sentient beings". All
this has led to an ethical reappraisal of animal experiments,
which helps to contribute to the search for a reduction in
numbers and/or refinement of experimental procedures, wherever
possible.
Table 10, chapter 5, concerning the distress aspect, showed that
the quality of vaccines in particular involves drastic
procedures. True, this research is aimed at the welfare of man

and animals so that, generally speaking, it will be justified on moral grounds. However, if we consider the quality control as having sprung from respect for life, then it will be clear that this view should also be extended to include the laboratory animal. Seen from this angle, the search for reduction and/or refinement of animal experiments in vaccine control deserves just as much our full attention.

2.2. Economic aspects

The requirements vaccines have to meet, and therefore the extent of the quality control, have become more stringent in the last few decades. Animal tests now account for a substantial proportion of the cost price of the vaccine product (for example, about 20% for the DPT vaccine) (3).

An added disadvantage of the animal experiment is that there may be a long time interval between the beginning and end of the experiment so that results are not immediately available, and this disrupts the continuity of the production and distribution process.

2.3. Zootechnical aspects

Working with living beings in an animal test implies that a variety of factors can influence the outcome and the reproducibility of an experiment. Table 1 gives a summary of these factors.

Stringent standardization of these factors (in which GMP plays an important part) and giving the experiment a statistical basis (among other things, by introducing a reference vaccine) can limit but not eliminate altogether the variability in the results. Unfortunately, these measures also raise the costs considerably.

2.4. Safety aspects

Despite the use of specific pathogen-free (SPF) animals (although not always possible) and working with colonies bred in the establishments' own laboratories, the experimental animal is -from a microbiological viewpoint - a potential risk factor, especially where live vaccines are produced. Viral contamination of the product can occur if cell cultures derived from infected animals are used for the production of vaccines. There is also the possibility of indirect contamination.

This was a serious problem in the production of inactivated polio vaccine in the recent past. The primary kidney cell cultures needed for its production were derived from imported monkeys caught in the wild. Many of these animals had contracted virus infections (13), including various semian viruses, such as SV40, or foamy virus. In most cases this led to rejection of the cell suspension (sometimes up to 50% of the suspensions) or of the vaccine product. This risk has decreased considerably over the last few years by using laboratory born and raised animals. Nevertheless, continual intensive serological monitoring of all animals - including SPF animals - required for vaccine production is still a stringent condition. This reduces the risk but does not fully exclude the likelihood of an infection.

Table 1: SUMMARY OF THE FACTORS THAT MAY INFLUENCE THE RESPONSE
OF THE EXPERIMENTAL ANIMAL (ADAPTED FROM STRASSER, 1973)
(4)

Factors	relevant literature on vaccine control
Physiological factors	
- age	Porter (5)
- sex	
- ovulation cycle	
- gestation and lactation	
- genetic variation	Pittman (6), Prigge (7)
- weight	
Environmental factors	
- environment:	
- temperature	Cameron (8)
- humidity	
- air (composition, flow)	
- light (intensity, quality, duration)	
- cage (size, material, shape)	
- bedding (type, amount, replacement)	
- handling (picking up, noise)	Porter (5)
- Hygiene:	
- macrobiological (animals in the cage, in the room)	
- microbiological (pathogenic and other microorganisms)	van Steenis (9) Abdussalam (10)
- Diet:	
- feed (composition, quantity, administration)	Knight (11) v.Ramshorst (12)
- drink (quality, quantity, administration)	
- Other:	
- transport	
- changes in the group/environment	
- acclimatization	

2.5. Practical aspects

The ability to detect undesirable particles (e.g. non-inactivated virus) in a vaccine liquid is related to the volume of the vaccine sample to be examined. Only small volumes can generally be tested by in vivo methods. In vitro tests have a larger capacity and are consequently usually more reliable. For this reason, the WHO Expert Group proposed in 1979 to replace the thus far officially prescribed test for residual live polio virus in monkeys with a tissue culture assay (15).
A special problem concerning animal tests is presented by the developing countries. Most of these countries have a high infant mortality rate, chiefly due to endemic infectious diseases, such as intestinal infections, measles, whooping cough and neonatal tetanus (16). The WHO has assigned high priority to combatting a number of these infectious diseases. To this end, the WHO

launched the "Expanded Programme on Immunization" (17), aimed particularly at the fight against diphtheria, tetanus, whooping cough, tuberculosis, poliomyelitis and measles by means of vaccination. Part of this programme is the planned production and control of vaccines at certain centres in developing countries. With the currently used methods, this will require many experimental animals in the near future, probably 2 to 5 times the present number (10, 18).

As regards the breeding of these animals, however, most developing countries contend with almost insurmountable problems, such as those connected with climatic conditions, genetic standardization and uniform feeding regimes. In addition, the costs of the experimental animals pose a problem, these often being much higher in the Third World than in Western countries. For these reasons the developing countries will benefit especially from simple tests requiring fewer animals, or from in vitro techniques.

As a result of the limitations outlined above, a growing interest can be observed in testing procedures which lead to the replacement, reduction or refinement of animal usage. These wishes can be fulfilled thanks to the current knowledge in the field of science and technology. Needless to say, animal experimentation has often been the basis for this development.

3. REFERENCES

1. CIOMS: Proposed International Guiding Principles for Biomedical Research Involving Animals. XVIIth CIOMS Round Table Conference, Geneva, Switzerland. 8-9 December 1983.
2. Osterhaus, A.D.M.E. and Steenis, G. van: Virologic control of monkeys used for the production of poliomyelitis vaccine. Develop. Biol. Standard. (1981), 47, 157-161.
3. Stainer, D.W. et al.: Reduction in animal usage for potency testing of diphtheria and tetanus toxoids. 19th IABS Congress on Use and Standardization of Combined Vaccines. Amsterdam, the Netherlands, 1985. Develop. Biol. Standard. (1986), 65, 241-244.
4. Strasser, H.: The choice of animals for drug testing seen from genetic aspects. In: The laboratory animal in drug testing. 5th ICLA Symposium, Hannover, 1972. Gustav Fischer Verlag. Stuttgart, 1973.
5. Porter, G. and Festing, M.: Effects of daily handling and other factors on weight gain of mice from birth to six weeks of age. Lab. Anim. (1969), 3, 7-16.
6. Pittman, M. and Cox, C.B.: Pertussis vaccine testing forfreedom from toxicity. Applied Microbiol. (1965), 13, 447-456.
7. Knight, P.A. and Lucken, R.N.: The effects of laboratory animal diets on the potency tests of bacterial vaccines. Develop. Biol. Standard. 1980), 45, 143-149.
8. Cameron, J.: The influence of environment on the mouse weight-gain test for estimating the toxicity of Bordetella pertussis vaccines. Progr. Immunobiol. Standard. (1969), 3, 319-323.
9. Steenis, G. van et al.: Use of captive-bred monkeys for vaccine production. Develop. Biol. Standard. (1980), 45, 99-105.
10. Abdussalam, M.: Animals for biomedical research: perspective of developing countries. XVIIth CIOMS Round Table Conference, Geneva, Switzerland, 8-9 December 1983.
11. Prigge, R.: Diphtherie-Schutzimpfung mit hochaktiven Impfstoffen. (Diphtheria vaccination using highly potent vaccines.) Ergebnisse der Hygiene, (1939), 22, 1-63.
12. Ramshorst, J.D. van: The influence of external factors on immune response in animals. Proc. Symposium on Bacterial Vaccines (1971), 313-315.
13. Osterhaus, A.D.M.E. and Steenis, G. van: Virologic control of monkeys used for the production of poliomyelitis vaccine. Develop. Biol. Standard. (1981), 47, 157-161.
14. Beale, A.J.: Cell substrate for killed polio-vaccine production. Develop. Biol. Standard. (1981), 47, 19-23.
15. Hennessen, W.: Replacement of animals in manufacture and control of vaccines. Develop. Biol. Standard. (1980), 45, 163-173.
16. Walsh, J.A. and Warren, K.S.: Selective primary health care. New. Engl. J. Med. (1979), 301, 967-974.
17. Keja, K. and Henderson, R.H.: Expanded Programme on Immunization: the continuing role of the European region. WHO Chronicle, (1985), 39, 3, 92-94.
18. Perkins, F.T.: The need for quality control in the developing countries. Develop. Biol. Standard. (1978), 41, 291-294.

CHAPTER 7: ALTERNATIVES TO AND IN ANIMAL EXPERIMENTATION

The growing interest in research techniques which lead to the
replacement, reduction or refinement of animal usage was pointed
out in the previous chapter. This interest can be noted
particularly in vaccine research. The WHO (1) and the European
Pharmacopoeia (2), among others, recognize the need for
developing so-called "alternative methods". This is the term
reserved for the above-mentioned research techniques and which
has the most widespread acceptance. In the following sections
attention will be paid to various aspects concerning
alternatives: definition, history, possiblities and lines of
approach.

1. DEFINITION

The "alternatives" concept frequently gives rise to a semantic
babel, although it is not entirely without reason.
Linguistically, an alternative is the choice between two things
or propositions. Applied to animal experimentation, it is the
choice between the classical animal experiment and another
(animal-sparing) method.
Many of the currently known alternatives do not meet this
definition, either because they do not replace the animal
experiment but only complement it (in this case it would be
better to speak of complementary or additional tests), or because
they are qualitatively better than the original animal test and
in this case introduction of an "alternative" is not a choice but
a scientific necessity. The use of cell cultures in the test for
foreign viruses in live vaccines can be regarded as an example of
a complementary test; the use of cell cultures for testing for
the presence of residual live viruses in the inactivated polio
vaccine is an example of a scientific necessity.
Although linguistically debatable, many misunderstandings can be
avoided by starting from the definition formulated by Smyth in
1978 (3): "Alternatives include any procedures which do away with
the use of animals altogether, lead to a reduction in the total
number of animals used, or lead to less distress to the animals
employed". This definition implies that complementary tests
should not be counted as alternative methods, while on the other
hand a reduction in the number of times blood is taken in a test
is a real alternative. Smyth based his definition on the
recommendations made by Russell and Burch (1959) to reduce
inhumanity in animal experimentation. These recommendations,
published in their book: "Principles of Humane Experimental
Technique" (4) have become known as the three Rs - Replacement,
Reduction and Refinement of animal usage. In a later phase the
concepts of Reason and Responsibility were added in order to
underline the essential role of the animal experimenter in this
pursuit.
(Note: A sixth R could be added to these five Rs, namely, the R
of Removal. As it will become clear later, it will be possible in
a few cases - albeit only under certain conditions - to drop an
animal test without its replacement by another procedure).
As regards an alternative, the following interpretation is given
by Smyth to the 3 Rs of Russell and Burch:
- replacement: replacement of higher animals by invertebrate
                organisms or non-biological material;

- reduction: the reduction in the number of animals required to
               solve a scientific problem;
- refinement: the reduction of stressful procedures in an animal
               experiment.

It should be noted that any "alternative" must provide results or
information which allow the same conclusions to be drawn with the
same degree of confidence.

Smyth's definition of the term "alternatives" applies whenever it
is used in this report.

2. HISTORY

The interest in alternatives in animal research is often regarded
as a feature of our time, but this representation is not entirely
correct. Although under a different name, the interest in
alternative techniques may be traced back many years. The
underlying idea was scientific or economic rather than ethical.
The traditional relationship between vaccine research and
experimental animal was pointed out in chapter 3. In a certain
sense this relationship also exists between vaccine research and
the development of alternatives. A few examples can elucidate
this.

One of the first alternative techniques described (1881) is
perhaps the application of agar-agar for the culture of bacteria.
Before that, potato slices or animals were used for this purpose.
Robert Koch's - accidental - discovery that agar gave better
results made the in vivo culture of bacteria less important.
Another "historical" alternative has already been described in
detail in chapter 3. In 1923 Ramon (5) developed an in vitro
method (the Lf determination) to replace the in vivo potency
assay of the tetanus and diphtheria vaccines.

Although the method proved to be unsuitable for the control of
the final product, it is still the official test used for the in-
process control of vaccine products. However, the major
developments in the past were in the field of viral vaccine
production (table 1).

Table 1: PRODUCTION TECHNIQUES FOR VIRAL VACCINES: REPLACEMENT OF
        IN VIVO CULTURE BY IN VITRO CULTURE (A FEW EXAMPLES)

Vaccine	In vivo	In vitro
Rabies	rabbit/mouse/sheep/ goat (brains)	primary dog kidney cells
Smallpox	calf (skin)	primary rabbit kidney cells
Mumps	monkey (salivary glands)	chick embryo fibroblasts
Foot-and-mouth disease	ox (tongue)	baby hamster kidney cells

The research of Woodruff and Goodpasture (6) into the use of
embryonated (hen) eggs (1931) and that of Enders (7) into the
application of cell cultures for growing the polio virus (1949)
have been of fundamental importance.
The development of an alternative to an existing method can be a
stepwise process, as will become clear from a closer
consideration of the production of inactivated polio vaccine.
Since Ender's discovery that polio vaccine virus could be
cultured in non-neuronal cells, and primary monkey kidney cells
were chosen for this purpose, there have been four developments
in this field which can all be regarded as alternatives:
a. improvement of the kidney perfusion and cell trypsinization
   techniques, enabling a substantial increase in the cell yield
   per kidney (8);
b. substitution of laboratory born and raised animals for
   imported monkeys caught in the wild. Since imported animals
   were frequently found to have contracted various virus
   infections (for example, with SV40 or foamy virus), the
   utilization of wild caught monkeys often led to contamination
   and rejection of the kidney cells obtained (sometimes up to
   50% (9, 10)). Few extraneous agents have been isolated from
   primary kidney cell cultures from animals bred in captivity
   under controlled conditions (11);
c. introduction of the microcarrier principle, so that the
   capacity of the virus culture could be greatly increased (12);
d. substitution of subcultured (tertiary) monkey kidney cells for
   primary monkey kidney cells. This made it possible to increase
   considerably the production of virus per kidney.
The impact of the introduction of these alternatives on the
number of monkeys required in the Netherlands is shown in table
2.

Table 2: ALTERNATIVES IN THE PRODUCTION OF INACTIVATED POLIO
         VACCINE AND THEIR EFFECT ON ANIMAL USE IN THE
         NETHERLANDS

year	technique	number of monkeys/year in the Netherlands
1960		2440
1965		4570
	in situ trypsinization	
1970		1590
	microcarrier technique	
1975		463
	use of monkeys from own breeding units	
1980	use of tertiary cell cultures	47
1984		30
	use of cell lines (?)	

Note: The polio vaccine was included in the DPT-polio
      immunization programme in 1962. The total production of
      polio vaccine in 1984 was roughly the same as that in 1965.

Paradoxically, the introduction of an alternative method does not always save animals. For example, there may be a shift within _in vivo_ research, or the introduction of a new _in vivo_ test may be necessary so that the total number of animals required is on balance increased. The substitution of tertiary monkey kidney cells for primary ones is a vivid example of this. On the one hand, this meant a fall in the number of monkeys required to serve as a donor animal but, on the other hand, it added a new _in vivo_ test to the quality control - the tumourigenicity test in rats - to detect possible oncogenic properties of serially propagated cells.

3. POSSIBILITIES

Some authors assign a limited value to alternative methods and consider their prospects rather gloomy because these alternatives ignore the complexicity of the intact organism. It is difficult to replace essential processes such as homeostasis, interaction between organ systems, metabolism and immune response by alternatives, and this fact makes the whole organism indispensable (13).
This statement seems to be inconsistent with the (potential) possibilities of alternative methods in vaccine production and control. What are the reasons for this? First, with several animal models used in the quality control of vaccines, relatively well-defined questions have to be answered, so that an integrated functioning of the different organ systems in the body is not strictly essential. Such tests are eminently suitable for _in vitro_ techniques, as is exemplified by the specific-toxicity test and the test for residual live virus. True, in a number of cases the knowledge to undertake the practical development of alternatives is still lacking. This is true, for example, of the potency assay on the tetanus vaccine. For those tests in which inter-systemic reactions can play a role such as, for example, the abnormal-toxicity and safety tests, the prospects for the development of _in vitro_ tests are not yet very promising.
The term "alternatives" is sometimes also misinterpreted as being solely a synonymn for an _in vitro_ technique. As stated in the introduction to this chapter, the term "alternatives" includes any technique leading to the replacement, reduction and/or refinement of animal usage. According to this definition, an alternative need not a priori replace an animal experiment entirely. An example is the decrease in the monkeys required for polio vaccine production as a result of substituting captive-bred animals for imported wild-caught ones.
An _in vitro_ test can also form part of an animal test, thereby taking over certain procedures in it. In many instances this makes it possible to reduce the number of animals needed or to make refinements in the technique used. Such opportunities also exist within the quality control. This is exemplified by the potency test on the diphtheria vaccine, where the lethal challenge was replaced by determination of the serum antibody titre using tissue culture. However, it should be borne in mind and this is true in general - that research on animals is often essential before _in vitro_ techniques can be developed, among other reasons, to validate research.

4. APPROACH

As part of the project an inventory has been made of the
possibilities of alternative methods (that is, methods which
differ from the existing ones in that they make it possible to
realize one or more of the Rs) in the production and control of
human and veterinary vaccines. The relevant literature and our
own research was consulted for this purpose. The results are
given in chapters 8 to 12 inclusive. The following three
approaches were taken for this survey:
- an evaluative approach, based on an analysis of the existing
  animal tests. Using information provided by the literature, the
  experts consulted, and our own investigation, recommendations
  are also made on how to modify existing animal tests with
  regard to reduction and refinement. As part of this approach
  the vaccine guidelines were catalogued, comparing national and
  international guidelines. The WHO guidelines (up to 1988), the
  European Pharmacopoeia guidelines (up to 1988), the UK
  guidelines (Britisch Pharmacopoeia, up to 1981/1985; White
  Book,up to 1978), the US guidelines (FDA, up to 1983), the
  Japanese guidelines (Minimum Requirements, up to 1983) and the
  Dutch specifications (up to 1988) were consulted.
- an innovative approach, with reference to the possibilities of
  achieving a replacement, reduction or refinement in the
  production and control of vaccines by means of new techniques.
  A summary is given of recent developments in this field. In
  addition, the results are given of a study conducted as part of
  this project on the opportunities to reduce the number of
  animals used in the potency test on the tetanus and diphtheria
  vaccines.
- an indirect approach, that is, changing the conditions under
  which the test is performed, so that the number of animals used
  can be reduced without altering the design and experimental
  procedure of the animal test. Several suggestions are
  discussed.
Although every attempt has been made to cover the subject as
completely as possible, this can never be fully accomplished in
such a large research field as the production and control of
vaccines.

62

5. REFERENCES

1. Anonymous: Report on an informal consultation on the assay of diphtheria and tetanus toxoids. Geneva, 12-14 December 1983.
2. Estoppey-Stojanowski, L.: Council of Europe Policy on Protection of Animals. Develop. Biol. Standard. (1986), 64, 3-5.
3. Smyth, D.H.: Alternatives to animal experiments. ScolarPress, London (1978), ISBN 0 85967 396 0.
4. Russell, W.M.S. and Burch, R.L.: Principles of Humane Experimental Technique. Methuen (1959).
5. Ramon, G.: Flocculation in mixtures of anti-diphtheria serum and toxin. Annales de l'Intitut Pasteur, (1923), 37, 12, 1001-1011.
6. Woodruff, A.M. and Goodpasture, E.W.: Susceptibility of chorio-allantoic membrane of chick embryos to infection with fowl-pox virus. Am. J. Path. (1931), 7, 209-222.
7. Enders, J.F. et al.: Cultivation of the Lansing strain of poliomyelitis virus in cultures of various human embryonic tissues. Science, (1949), 247, 12, 1726-1728.
8. Kammer, H.: Cell dispersal methods for increasing yield from animal tissues. Applied Microbiology (1969), 17, 4, 524-527.
9. Steenis, G. van et al.: Use of captive-bred monkeys forvaccine production. Develop. Biol. Standard. (1979), 45, 99-105.
10. Beale, A.J.: Cell substrate for killed polio vaccine production. Develop. Biol. Standard. (1981), 47, 19-23.
11. W.H.O., Technical Report Series 687 (1983).
12. Wezel, A.L. van et al.: New approach to the production of concentrated and purified inactivated polio and rabies tissue culture vaccines. Develop. Biol. Standard. (1978), 41, 159-168.
13. Weihe, W.H.: Use and misuse of an imprecise concept: alternative methods in animal experiments. Lab. Anim. (1985), 19, 19-26.

CHAPTER 8: OPPORTUNITIES FOR REPLACEMENT, REDUCTION OR REFINEMENT: HUMAN BACTERIAL VACCINES

1. INTRODUCTION

This chapter reviews the six bacterial* vaccines produced in the Netherlands for routine use. They are also used worldwide. They are:
- BCG vaccine;
- cholera vaccine;
- diphtheria vaccine;
- pertussis vaccine;
- tetanus vaccine;
- typhoid vaccine.

The diphtheria, pertussis and tetanus vaccines are included in the National Vaccination Programme. Because of this, the annual volume produced for these vaccines (chapter 5, table 3) - and therefore also the number of animals required - is considerably higher than for the other products.

In general more experimental animals are used in the quality control of human bacterial vaccines than in that of viral vaccines. Important tests in this connection are the potency assay and the test for specific toxicity.

The types of control tests and the opportunities for using alternative methods are given for each vaccine in the following table.

Abnormal toxicity test	Skin reactivity test	Potency test	Specific-toxicity test	Identity test	
±	±	0	-	0	BCG vaccine
0	-	-	±	+	Cholera vaccine
0	±	+	±	+	Diphtheria vacc.
0	±	-	-	0	Pertussis vaccine
0	±	+	±	+	Tetanus vaccine
0	-	-	-	+	Typhoid vaccine

Key
0: The test is not stipulated or is based on an in vitro method;
-: The in vivo test is statutory; according to the author, there is at present no possibility of replacement, reduction or refinement in the use of laboratory animals;
±: An alternative approach to the test is described, but it still needs validation and/or discussion in a broader context;
+: An alternative approach to the test is described, which can be used as such, or which already finds application.

---

* The Haemophilus influenzae vaccine will be added to this range of products in the near future.

2. BCG VACCINE

The BCG vaccine (abbreviation of Bacille Calmette Guérin) is a
freeze-dried live bacterial vaccine which is used for active
immunization against tuberculosis and also - on a limited scale -
as an immunological adjuvant in the treatment of patients with
tumours.
The following animal tests are relevant to its quality control:
- test for absence or virulent mycobacteria;
- skin reactivity, or Jensen test;
- test for abnormal toxicity.

2.1. <u>Test for absence of virulent mycobacteria</u>
The BCG vaccine contains an attenuated Mycobacterium strain. To
check that no virulent bacteria are present, guinea pigs are
inoculated subcutaneously with several times the human dose,
followed by an observation period of 6 weeks. None of the animals
should show any signs of tuberculosis during this period and no
more than one animal is allowed to die from a cause other than
tuberculosis.
Table 1 summarizes the existing guidelines and their
specifications for this test.

Table 1: THE GUIDELINES AND THEIR SPECIFICATIONS FOR THE TEST FOR
         ABSENCE OF VIRULENT MYCOBACTERIA

Specifications	\multicolumn{6}{c}{Distress category 1*}					
	WHO (1)	Eur.Ph. (2)	Neth. (3)	UK (4)	USA (5)	Japan (6)
Species	guinea pig	guinea pig	guinea pig	guinea pig	guinea pig	guinea pig
No. of animal groups	1	1	1	1	1	1
No. of animals/ group	≥ 6	6	6	6	≥ 6	6
Route of administration	s.c./ i.m.	s.c.	s.c. i.m.	s.c.	s.c./ i.m.	s.c./ i.m.
Observation period	≥ 6 wk.	≥ 6 wk.	≥ 6 wk.	≥ 6 wk.	6 wk.	3 m.
Criterion	\multicolumn{6}{c}{.......... Tuberculosis-free ....}					

* See chapter 5, section 4.
s.c. = subcutaneous;   i.m. = intramuscular;
wk. = weeks;   m.   = months.

There is broad agreement on the number of animals, route of
administration and length of the observation period. There are at
present no possibilities for replacement, reduction or
refinement. However, there are indications that it might be
possible to distinguish between virulent and nonvirulent germs on
the basis of a bacteriological test.

2.2. Jensen test (skin reactivity test)

The BCG strains currently in use react differently after
intracutaneous administration. If the vaccine produces too strong
a response, it can lead to severe local reactions in the
vaccinees. Therefore, the reactivity of the final product is
determined, usually in comparison with a reference vaccine of
known (acceptable) reactivity in children and adults.
The guinea pig serves as a model. The procedure is as follows:
several dilutions of the vaccine to be tested and of the
reference preparation are injected intradermally at various
sites, and the resulting skin reaction (redness, swelling) is
subsequently read at different times thereafter. The test vaccine
should not produce a skin reaction that is significantly stronger
than that caused by the reference vaccine. Table 2 lists the
existing guidelines and their specifications for this test.

Table 2: THE GUIDELINES AND THEIR SPECIFICATIONS FOR THE JENSEN
TEST

| Specifications | Distress category 4* | | | | | |
	WHO (1)	Eur.Ph. (2)	Neth. (3)	UK (4)	USA (5)	Japan (6)
Species	guinea pig	guinea pig	guinea pig	guinea pig	guinea pig	guinea pig
No. of animal groups	1	1	1	1	1	1
No. of animals/ group	≥ 4	2	6	2	≥ 2	6
Route of administration	i.d.	i.d.	i.d.	i.d.	i.d.	i.d.
No. of injections	6	6	6	6	4	n.s.
Reference vaccine	yes	yes	yes	yes	no	yes
Observation period	4 wk.	n.s.	5 w.k.	n.s.	n.s.	n.s.
Criterion	.... Skin reactions					

* See chapter 5, section 4.
i.d. = intradermal;   n.s. = not specified

The Dutch guidelines' specifications differ from those of the
other guidelines as regards the number of animals required. This
discrepancy results from a difference in the testing procedure.
In the Netherlands, two vaccine products are tested
simultaneously, that is, each animal receives 2 dilutions of each
of two vaccine products and 2 dilutions of the reference product
(a total of 6 injections). The other guidelines are based on 3
dilutions of one test vaccine and 3 dilutions of the reference
preparation per test.
The Dutch specifications could be brought into line with those of
the European Pharmacopoeia by reducing the number of animals to 4
while retaining the procedure used, but little would be gained by
this. Moreover, the outcome of the test differs considerably as a
result of the subjectivity of the assessment criterion. The
American guidelines do not mention a reference preparation.
However, the use of such a preparation is advisable on account of
the individual sensivity of the animals.

2.3. Test for abnormal toxicity

Since testing for abnormal toxicity forms part of the quality
control of all human vaccines, the particulars of this test given
in this section apply not only to the BCG vaccine but also to the
other vaccines to be discussed in this and in the following
chapter.
The last stage of the production process of all vaccines is the
filling of vials or ampoules with the final product. The purpose
of the abnormal-toxicity test is to detect any possible
(chemical) contamination of the product during this stage. To
that end, 2 guinea pigs and 5 mice are injected intraperitoneally
or subcutaneously with the final product, followed by an
observation period of 7 days. The animals are weighed just before
inoculation and at the end of the observation period.
The experiment is repeated if one or more of the following
criteria are not met:
- all the animals survived the observation period;
- none of the animals showed any weight loss at the end of the
  observation period;
- none of the animals showed toxic signs.
If after the first repeat these criteria are still not met, the
test is repeated a second time but now with twice as many
animals.
Table 3 summarizes the existing guidelines and their
specifications. It reveals considerable uniformity, except for
the number of animals used. The choice of two animal species is
based on the - empirical - assumption that the likelihood of
detecting a toxic effect increases when more animal species are
used, in this case, one rodent and one non-rodent.

Table 3: THE GUIDELINES AND THEIR SPECIFICATIONS FOR THE ABNORMAL
TOXICITY TEST (GENERAL)

| Specifications | Distress category 1* | | | | | |
	WHO (7)	Eur.Ph. (8)	Neth. (3)	UK (4)	USA (5)	Japan (6)
Species	guinea pig + mouse	guinea pig + mouse	guinea pig + mouse	guinea pig + mouse	guinea pig + mouse	guinea pig + mouse
No. of animals	≥2 g.p. ≥5 mice	2 g.p. 5 mice	2 g.p. 5 mice	2 g.p. 5 mice	≥2 g.p. ≥2 mice	2 g.p. 2 mice
Route of administration	s.c./ i.p.	s.c./ i.p.	s.c./ i.p.	s.c./ i.p.	s.c./ i.p.	s.c./ i.p.
Observation period (days)	7	7	7	7	7	7
Criteria	.... Weight loss + toxic signs					

* See chapter 5, section 4
g.p. = guinea pigs;   s.c. = subcutaneous;
i.p. = intraperitoneal.

The abnormal-toxicity test is currently under discussion (9) for
the following reasons:
- the importance of the test has been considerably diminished by
  the introduction of Good Manufacturing Practice (GMP) and
  chemical control tests;

- the test is of an aspecific nature; results are difficult to
  extrapolate to man because of the poor correlation with
  reactions occurring in man;
- this test is not mandatory for most of the pharmaceutical
  products;
- the test can only detect serious calamities giving rise to
  acute effects.

A suvey was made of the results of abnormal-toxicity tests
performed within the National Institute of Public Health and
Environmental Protection (RIVM) in the Netherlands during the
period 1982-1986 (table 4). It gives an impression of the
relevance of this test.

Table 4: SURVEY OF THE ABNORMAL-TOXICITY TEST ON HUMAN VACCINES,
         1982-1986 (RIVM)

Total No. of tests for abnormal toxicity, 1982-1986	753
The number of tests not meeting the requirements being	44
of which on: - mice	12
- guinea pigs	31
- mice + guinea pigs	1
1st Repeats	44
The number of tests not meeting the requirements being	3
of which on: - mice	1
- guinea pigs	2
2nd Repeats	3
The number of tests not meeting the requirements being	1
namely, on mice	1

The total number of vaccines rejected in the Netherlands between
1982 and 1986 because of abnormal toxicity was thus only 1.
Closer examination of the data on this vaccine batch suggests
that the reasons for rejection was not related to the vaccine
product itself but to other, fortuitous, circumstances.
The only conclusion to be drawn from the above data is that the
cause of nonfulfilment of the requirements is nearly always
aspecific. However, it does not furnish proof that the test is
unnecessary. Still, it seems justified to review the guidelines
for the abnormal-toxicity test. For example, a reduction in the
number of animals to two guinea pigs and two mice could be
considered in the first instance, in accordance with the Japanese
requirements. In addition, it may be questioned how much the
relevance of the test for abnormal toxicity is increased by using
a second animal species. It does not (yet) seem feasible to
dispense with the test, but this may become possible after a
complete validation of the GMP requirements for the packaging
process. At a recent international forum (9) it emerged that most
manufacturers want to retain the test because of possible
liability suits, among other reasons. They are prepared, however,
to increase the capacity of the vessels from which the vials and
ampoules are filled, thereby reducing the number of abnormal-
toxicity tests that need to be performed.

3. CHOLERA VACCINE

The cholera vaccine is a bivalent, inactivated product, prepared
from equal quantities of an Inaba and an Ogawa bacterial
suspension. It should be mentioned that the mode of action of the
cholera vaccine is still open to question. The following quality
control tests are relevant as regards the objectives of this
project:
- identity test;
- test for specific toxicity;
- endotoxin test (not stipulated officially);
- potency test;
- test for abnormal toxicity.

3.1. Identity test
The WHO guidelines (7) mention an *in vivo* test as one of the ways
to establish identity, without giving a specification for this.
In the Dutch specifications the identity test is based on an *in
vitro* assay (agglutination).

3.2. Test for specific toxicity
In general, the animal model used for this purpose is based on
the same principle as the test for abnormal toxicity. Animals are
injected intraperitoneally and observed for a few days.
Assessment is made on the basis of weight loss and clinical signs
and symptoms. The existing guidelines show little uniformity (see
table 5). The WHO, the European Pharmacopoeia and the British
Pharmacopoeia have no guidelines for this test.
There is agreement on the use of the mouse as the test animal and
on the mode of administration. The specifications differ as
regards the use of the guinea pig as a model, the number of
animals and the length of the observation period.
Cholera does not cause any specific symptoms in mice and guinea
pigs, and this necessitates an extensive examination of the
vaccine for abnormal toxicity.
Since the specific toxicity test is combined with the test for
abnormal toxicity, it seems unwise to dispense with the guinea
pig as a model. A reduction of the number of mice to about 5 may
be possible.

Table 5: THE EXISTING GUIDELINES AND THEIR SPECIFICATIONS FOR THE
SPECIFIC TOXICITY TEST ON CHOLERA VACCINE

| Specifications | Distress category 1* | | |
	Neth.(3)	USA(5)	Japan (6)
Species	guinea pig + mouse	mouse	mouse
No. of animals	3 guinea pigs + 10 mice	10-40	5
Route of administration	i.p.	i.p.	i.p.
Observation period	7 days	72 hr	72 hr
Criterion	.... body weight and clinical signs		

* See chapter 5, section 4
i.p. = intraperitoneal

3.3. Endotoxin test

Endotoxins are lipopolysaccharide complexes present in the outer coating of gram-negative bacteria. These components can occur in the vaccine either in the free form or - in the case of vaccines made from gram-negative bacteria - bound to the bacterial cell wall. Parenteral administration of such a product causes a rise in body temperature.

In the past, the presence of endotoxins was established by the pyrogenicity test, requiring at least 3 rabbits. This test involved recording the body temperature for at least 3 hours following parenteral administration of the product to be examined. Despite the limitations of its laborious nature, and also of the biological variability of the animals (10), the pyrogenicity test proved to be a reliable method. There is now an alternative method for demonstrating endotoxins, the Limulus amoebocyte lysate (LAL) test, an in vitro assay described by Levin in 1964 (11). The test makes use of the property of amoebocyte lysate (an extract prepared from the blood cells (amoebocytes) of the horseshoe crab* (Limulus polyphemus)) to form a gel in the presence of endotoxins. There are now several ways of carrying out the LAL test, all similar as regards the operating principle but differing in the method of determination (10, 13).

Since the various Limulus lysate products differ in biological activity, it is advisable to include a reference endotoxin in the test (14). Both the FDA and the WHO have a standard preparation for this purpose. The European Pharmacopoeia standard will be available shortly, after publication of a monograph on the LAL-test.

The LAL test is a cheap and reliable method for human vaccines. (Note: testing for endotoxin is not statutory for bacterial vaccine control.)

3.4. Potency test

There are no animal species which are naturally susceptible to infection by cholera vibrions. The current models for the potency test are therefore highly artificial. Table 6 lists the guidelines and their specifications for this test.

---

* To obtain the blood cells, the crab is captured, blood is withdrawn and the animal is then returned to the water; 90 per cent of the animals survive this operation (12).

Table 6: THE GUIDELINES AND THEIR SPECIFICATIONS FOR THE POTENCY
TEST ON CHOLERA VACCINE

Specifications	WHO (7)	Eur.Ph. (15)	Neth. (3)	USA (5)	Japan (6)
		Distress category 1*			
Species	mouse	guinea pig/ rabbit/ mouse	rabbit	mouse	mouse
No. of animal groups	3	n.s.	1	4	3
No. of animals/ group	15	≥6	3	16	10
Route of administration	s.c./ i.p.	n.s.	i.v.(4x)	i.p.	i.p.
Duration:					
-immunization (days)	7-14		15	12-16	12-16
-assessment after challenge (hours)	72		n.s.	48	72
Reference vaccine	yes			yes	yes
-no. of animal groups	3			4	n.s.
Control group	yes,4			yes,4	yes,3
-no. of animals/ group	10			10	10
Mode of challenge	i.p.			i.p.	i.p.
Criterion	death	serum titre	serum titre	death	death

* See chapter 5, section 4 (applies only to the Dutch
  specifications).
n.s. = not specified;   s.c. = subcutaneous;
i.v. = intravenous;   i.p. = intraperitoneal.

This table shows that there are large differences as regards both
design and execution of this test, which can be partly ascribed
to the contradictory data on the correlation between the potency
of the vaccine found from animal studies and its efficacy in
human field trials (16).
It can be concluded that to date there is no suitable animal
model available for potency testing of this vaccine. Any test
involving many animals is consequently irrelevant.
A new method currently being validated is the so-called DISC
model (17). Vaccinated rabbits are challenged locally with a
virulent cholera strain in the duodenum (DI). At the same time
the ileum (S) is ligated temporarily to enable the cholera
bacteria to colonize the duodenum, and the coecum (C) is ligated
permanently to prevent resorption of the fluid secreted by the
small intestine. The preliminary results indicate that this model
may hold better prospects from a scientific point of view. Since
this test is highly stressful to the animals, a number of aspects
merit particular attention during its development phase, such as
the possibility of using postoperative anaesthesia or the use of
analgesic agents, of refining the procedure and of developing an
in vitro system based on this in vivo test.

3.5. Test for abnormal toxicity
See Section 2.3. of this chapter.

4. DIPHTHERIA VACCINE

The detoxified toxin (the toxoid) of Corynebacterium diphtheriae, often supplemented with an adjuvant, is used for active immunization purposes. Vaccination against diphtheria occurs worldwide. As regards the objectives of the present project - the 3 Rs - the following tests are important in the quality control of this product:
- identity test;
- test for specific toxicity;
- potency test;
- test for abnormal toxicity.

4.1. Identity test

There are both in vivo and in vitro methods for this test. The European Pharmacopoeia stipulates an in vivo test, while the WHO guidelines offer the user the choice between an in vivo test and several in vitro assays.
The in vivo method has several drawbacks; it requires animals, is expensive and time-consuming. In vitro methods do not have these disadvantages and they are moreover reliable, so that they are preferable to the in vivo test (18). These in vitro methods are usually based on precipitation of the toxoid with antitoxin. The flocculation, the single radial immunodiffusion (SRD) and the double immunodiffusion (DD) assays all find application.

4.2. Test for specific toxicity

A toxic product is obtained if the diphtheria toxin is not completely inactivated. This can be demonstrated by the specific-toxicity test. This test consists of inoculating a group of guinea pigs subcutaneously with an excess of the vaccine product, followed by an observation period of about 5 to 6 weeks. Depending on its concentration, the presence of non-inactivated toxin leads to results ranging from death within 12 hours (high toxin concentration) to progressive paralysis of the animals after 10 to 14 days (low toxin concentration). The test is performed both on the unpurified product during in-process control and on the purified toxoid and the adsorbed vaccine in the final control. Table 7 summarizes the existing guidelines and their specifications for the testing of the final product.

Table 7: EXISTING GUIDELINES AND THEIR SPECIFICATIONS FOR THE SPECIFIC-TOXICITY TEST ON THE DIPHTHERIA VACCINE

Specifications	WHO (1)	Eur.Ph. (19)	Neth. (3)	UK (4)	Japan (6)
		Distress category 1-4*			
Species	guinea pig	guinea pig	guinea pig	guinea pig	guinea pig
No. of animal groups	1	1	1	1	1
No. of animals/group	≥ 5	5	5	5	≥ 4
Route of administration	s.c.	s.c.	s.c.	s.c.	s.c.
Observation period	6 wk	6 wk	6 wk	30 d	30 d
Criterion	.... diphtheria symptoms				

* See chapter 5, section 4;   s.c. = subcutaneous

It shows that there is agreement on the mode of administration, the dose and the criterion applied. There are only small differences as regards the number of animals required and the length of the observation period. A slight reduction in the number of animals could be achieved by adopting the Japanese guidelines. Another approach is to reduce the number of in-process quality control tests of vaccine batches. Thorough experience with the process of detoxifying the diphtheria toxin and with diphtheria vaccine production, in accordance with general GMP principles and guidelines, may make it possible to restrict the test for specific toxicity to the purified product only.

An alternative, in vitro, method to the guinea pig model was described recently (20). This method is based on the determination of the residual toxicity in a tissue culture system. Increasing dilutions of the vaccine product are added to cultures of Vero cells in microtitre plates. The plates are assessed on the basis of cytotoxic reactions. A good statistical correlation was found to exist between the in vitro and the in vivo method. Compared with the guinea pig model, this in vitro method is not only an attractive alternative from an ethical viewpoint but it is also sensitive, reproducible, cheap and takes only 72 hours to complete (as opposed to 30 days for the guinea pig model). This offers many advantages particularly for in-process control.

The results of a validation currently being undertaken by the RIVM confirm the conclusions made about the control of the purified toxoid (21).

The unpurified product interferes with the cell culture, probably because of contaminants in the product, for instance, medium components, formaldehyde, etc. This requires further investigation. It can be concluded that the Vero-cell assay is a valuable alternative to the guinea pig model, at least for testing of the final product.

4.3. Potency test

There are several methods available for testing the efficacy of the diphtheria vaccine. The "in vitro" techniques described in this connection are based on the determination of either antigen (e.g. the flocculation test) or diphtheria antitoxin (e.g. heamagglutination and a Toxoid-ELISA assay). The problem with the former is that there is frequently no correlation between the amount of antigen and its protective action, which is partly due to variable factors such as the immunopotentiating activity of the adjuvant added and route of administration. The Toxoid-ELISA and haemagglutinin assays are generally not considered to be appropriate substitutes for animal test systems for two reasons. One reason is that animals are still needed for immunization purposes, and the other is that the Toxoid-ELISA and the haemagglutination tests cannot discriminate between neutralizing and non-neutralizing antibodies (22). This means that for the time being in vivo challenge models will have to be used.

Table 8 summarizes the guidelines and their specifications for this test.

The table shows that there are marked differences between the American guidelines and the others. The former are based on a qualitative assay, the requirement being that the toxoid is capable of inducing a defined antitoxin titre in experimental animals.

Table 8: THE GUIDELINES AND THEIR SPECIFICATIONS FOR THE POTENCY
TEST.

Specifications	WHO[***] (1)	Eur.Ph. (19)	Distress category 4* Neth. (3)	UK (4)	USA[**] (23)	Japan[***] (6)
species	guinea pig	guinea pig	guinea pig	guinea pig	guinea pig	guinea pig
No.of animal groups	3	3	3	3	1	n.s.
No. of animals/ group	n.s.	16	20	16	4	10
Route of administration	s.c.	s.c.	s.c.	s.c.	s.c.	s.c.
Duration: -immunization (days)	28	28	28	28	n.s.	28-42
-assessment after challenge (days)	5	4	4	4		7
No. of control groups	5	4	3	n.s.	1	3
Reference vaccine	yes	yes	yes	yes	no	yes
-no. of animal group	3	3	3	3		n.s.
-no. of animals/ group	n.s.	16	20	16		
Mode of challenge	s.c.	s.c.	s.c.	s.c.	serum	n.s.
Criterion	death	death	death	death	titration in 4 g.p.	death

* See chapter 5, section 4
** US requirements for adsorbed diphtheria toxoid.
*** Both the Japanese and the latest (34) WHO guidelines state
   that the antitoxin titration method may be used as an
   alternative to the in vivo test.
g.p. = guinea pigs;   s.c. = subcutaneous;   n.s. = not specified;

The other guidelines are based on a quantitative dose-response
assay in which 3 dilutions of the vaccine being examined are
compared with 3 dilutions of a reference preparation using a
lethal challenge test; the relative potency with 95% fudicial
limits is expressed in international units (I.U.). (This assay is
also called 3+3 assay, or parallel-line bioassay.) In practice,
the qualitative assay is very sensitive to various influences
(e.g. the animals are not equally susceptible to the test
substance). The introduction of a standard preparation can
increase the standardizability of the qualitative assay, making
it a useful model for routine efficacy testing. It is in any case
advisable to evaluate the usefulness of such a modified
qualitative assay (also called two-point method). Currently, the
quantitative method is generally preferred from a statistical
viewpoint. However, it suffers from two drawbacks (24):
- it requires large numbers of laboratory animals and the testing
  procedure causes much distress (category 4);
- it is also costly.

4.3.1. Alternative methods
One alternative is the multiple intradermal challenge test (25).
It differs from the above-mentioned method in that the lethal
challenge is replaced by an intradermal challenge with various
dilutions of the diphtheria toxin. Assessment takes place on the
basis of skin reactions. By assigning a score to these reactions,
the potency can be calculated in relation to that of a reference
preparation.
The advantage of the multiple intradermal challenge is that the
amount of information provided by each animal is greater than is
the case with the lethal challenge, so that fewer animals are
needed per vaccine dilution. In addition, the challenge inflicts
less stress on the animals (category 2). On the other hand,
disadvantages include the subjectivity of the assessment criteria
and the labour intensiveness of this method. This method has been
recognized for some years now by various regulatory bodies such
as the WHO and the European Pharmacopoeia Commission.
A second alternative approach for determining the efficacy of the
diphtheria vaccine has recently been developed (26) and validated
(27). In this method, the principle of which was described before
(28), the potency is no longer determined by means of a lethal or
intradermal challenge but by serum titration and neutralization
in tissue culture (Vero cells) (see chapter 3, section 5). This
model contributes to both a refinement of the experimental
procedure and a reduction in animals: the distress-causing
challenge is replaced by a combined exsanguination-euthanasia
procedure (distress category 1), and since each animal provides
more information, a considerable reduction in the number of
animals required can be achieved. This method has recently been
adopted by the Dutch control authorities and is mentioned in
small print in the latest WHO guidelines (34) on diphtheria
vaccine.

4.3.2. Reduction of group size
Table 8 shows that the WHO guidelines do not specify the number
of animals to be used for the lethal challenge test, but they do
recommend that the number of animals be sufficient to assure a
95% confidence interval within the range of 50-200% of the
estimated potency. The European Pharmacopoeia does not have this
requirement, but stipulates that the lower fiducial limit of the
estimated potency of the vaccine should exceed a specified number
of international units.
Although strictly speaking it was not one of the objectives of
this project, it was decided, in consultation with the RIVM, to
devote a part of the project period to examining the possibility
of reducing the number of laboratory animals for the efficacy
testing of the diphtheria vaccine, yet at the same time complying
with the requirements of the WHO guidelines and the European
Pharmacopoeia.
To this end, the author of this report made a computer study of
28 batches of diphtheria vaccine which had previously been
examined by the RIVM for their efficacy using the traditional
method (lethal challenge, 20 guinea pigs per dilution).
Hypothetical, random groups of 16, 14, 12, 10 and 8 animals per
vaccine dilution were set up using the original data. The potency
of the product and its 95% confidence interval were then
recalculated for the different group sizes. The results for the
DPT-polio (diphtheria, pertussis - whooping cough, tetanus,
poliomyelitis) batches are summarized in table 9.

As expected, the range of the 95% confidence interval increased with decreasing group size. To obtain an idea of the changes in this interval, the potency of each vaccine product was set at 100% and the upper and lower limits of the 95% confidence interval were expressed as a percentage of the potency. The results for the 28 diphtheria vaccine batches are shown in figure 1.

It can be deduced from table 9 and figure 1 that it is possible to reduce the size of the group to about 12 animals while still complying with the guidelines of the WHO and the European Pharmacopoeia (the lower limit being particularly important in the latter) (29). This finding agrees with the results of similar studies conducted concurrently in Britain (30, 31) and Canada (32).

On the basis of the Dutch, British and Canadian results, an informal working party submitted proposals (33) to the WHO in December 1985 concerning the use of experimental animals for the potency assay of diphtheria vaccines. The proposals were adopted in 1987 by the Expert Committee of the WHO (34) stating that when consistency of production and testing has been established, the minimum number of animals used per dilution of vaccine may be substantially decreased, for example halved, provided that the assays are statistically valid.

As part of the project the author made a similar computer analysis of the effect of group size on the potency and 95% confidence interval for the mouse model used to determine the potency of diphtheria vaccines (serum neutralization test). This model was originally based on 12 animals per vaccine dilution. The potency and the 95% confidence interval were recalculated for the diphtheria component of 17 vaccine batches from the data obtained on the animals. The results for these 17 batches are summarized in table 10, and figure 2 shows the effect of group size on the 95% confidence interval.

A reduction from 12 to 6 or 8 mice per vaccine dilution is acceptable if the WHO requirement (50-200% range) is implemented. A striking feature of the mouse model is that for groups of up to 6 animals per dilution the range of the 95% confidence interval is very small when compared with the lethal challenge test in guinea pigs.

4.3.3. <u>Summary of the opportunities for reducing the number of animals required for the potency testing of the diphtheria component in vaccines</u>

As regards the traditional potency assay of the diphtheria component in combined vaccines (that is, the lethal challenge procedure involving 16-20 animals per vaccine dilution) the following alternatives exist for reducing or refining the use of animals:

Alternative 1: the lethal challenge in guinea pigs, based on using 10-12 animals per vaccine dilution (distress category 4);

Alternative 2: the multiple intradermal challenge in guinea pigs, based on using about 8 animals per dilution (distress category 2);

Alternative 3: serum neutralization in VERO cells (the mouse model), based on using 6-8 mice per dilution (distress category 1).

Table 9: **THE EFFECT OF A REDUCTION IN THE NUMBERS OF ANIMALS ON THE ESTIMATE OF POTENCY AND THE 95%**
CONFIDENCE INTERVAL FOR 9 BATCHES DPT-POLIO VACCINE IN THE DIPHTHERIA LETHAL CHALLENGE TEST

	Number of guinea pigs per dilution and potency in IU/ml									
	20		16		14		12		10		8
Batch number*	IU/ml	95% interval	IU/ml	95% interval	IU/ml	95% interval	IU/ml	95% interval	IU/ml	95% interval	IU/ml	95% interval
DPT-polio 125	63.8	41- 99	65.0	37-113	63.9	34-116	62.5	31-121	49.6	17-104	40.4	8- 92
DPT-polio 126	72.2	55- 95	68.6	49- 96	64.6	44- 94	70.7	44-116	70.0	39-131	63.0	33-125
DPT-polio 127	98.2	74-131	93.6	66-132	97.0	65-143	101.8	68-155	102.3	63-173	110.5	50-219
DPT-polio 128	93.7	67-131	96.1	64-146	100.3	63-165	106.4	59-202	90.8	46-179	102.6	56-206
DPT-polio 129	103.7	77-141	103.4	73-149	102.3	69-154	107.7	65-168	108.0	61-201	122.7	53-828
DPT-polio 130	88.6	60-134	93.0	58-157	97.9	56-192	99.1	57-191	100.0	48-262	92.9	42-241
DPT-polio 131	69.9	49- 98	72.0	48-105	79.6	54-117	76.1	48-118	70.8	39-145	65.4	25-170
DPT-polio 132	90.4	65-129	78.0	54-114	74.5	48-114	84.7	53-139	69.6	42-112	65.4	38-108
DPT-polio 133	96.4	68-139	97.9	65-150	101.3	67-159	85.2	54-136	93.5	54-170	100.1	48-239

* D=Diphtheria,   P=Pertussis,   T=Tetanus
IU=International Units
European Pharmacopoeia requirement for DPT-polio $\geq$ 30 IU/ml

Table 10: **THE EFFECT OF A REDUCTION IN THE NUMBERS OF ANIMALS ON THE ESTIMATE OF POTENCY AND THE 95%**
CONFIDENCE INTERVAL FOR 17 BATCHES OF COMBINED VACCINE ESTIMATED WITH THE SERUM NEUTRALIZATION
TEST IN MICE

	Number of mice per dilution and potency in IU/ml								
	12		10		8		6		4	
Batch number*	IU/ml	95% interval	IU/ml	95% interval	IU/ml	95% interval	IU/ml	95% interval	IU/ml	95% interval
DPT-polio 302	202	146-296	186	127-279	206	135-327	175	110-287	145	87-252
DT -polio 65	15	10- 22	14	9- 20	13	9- 21	13	8- 20	14	7- 29
DPT-polio 128	92	64-136	82	56-123	90	58-143	79	50-129	69	41-124
DPT-polio 303	233	159-342	214	140-323	246	159-383	277	173-456	350	196-696
DT -polio 69	16	11- 23	16	11- 25	15	10- 24	15	10- 23	17	11- 26
DPT-polio 127	85	57-124	93	61-141	100	64-155	121	81-189	115	68-201
DPT 103	245	176-343	270	192-381	288	195-432	298	219-412	339	230-521
DT -polio 68	13	9- 18	13	9- 18	13	9- 19	**		12	6- 22
DPT-polio 126	113	81-158	99	71-139	114	77-170	129	89-190	128	78-221
DPT 104	233	153-357	256	162-410	244	152-393	286	175-480	284	158-542
DT -polio 71	19	12- 28	19	12- 30	16	10- 26	18	11- 30	18	9- 35
DPT-polio 130	74	62-143	98	62-155	97	61-156	120	74-201	97	41-233
DPT 107	293	201-447	277	191-413	280	187-433	283	172-486	316	188-599
DT -polio 67	14	9- 19	13	9- 19	15	10- 22	14	8- 22	14	6- 29
DPT 106	187	136-257	**		171	109-268	178	121-260	**	
DT -polio 72	13	9- 18	11	7- 16	15	9- 23	13	9- 19	13	6- 26
DPT-polio 131	75	55-103	73	50-108	90	58-141	85	58-124	131	62-386

* D=Diphtheria,   P=Pertussis,   T=Tetanus
** =No common b-slope
IU=International Units
European Pharmacopoeia requirement for DPT-polio $\geq$ 30 IU/ml, DT-polio $\geq$ 5 IU/ml, DPT $\geq$ 60 IU/ml.

Fig. 1:
95% Confidence interval as a function of the size of the groups
of guinea pigs used for each dilution in the potency assay on the
diptheria component in vaccines

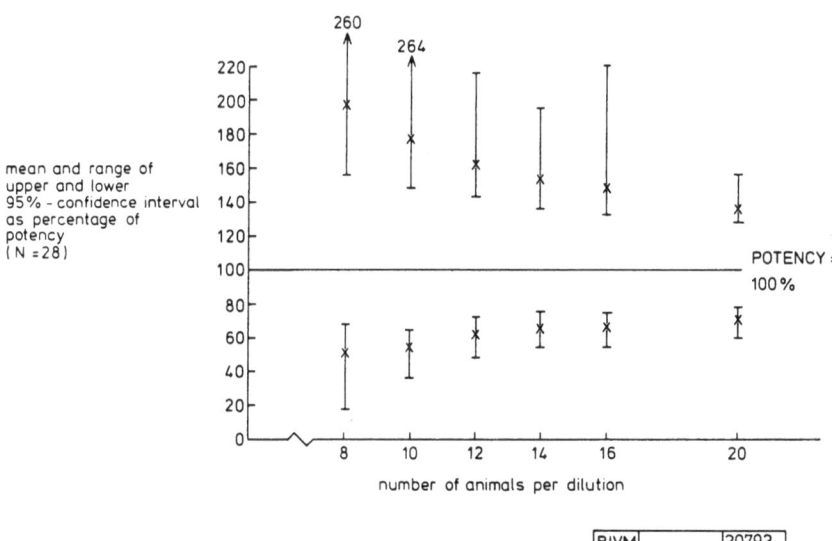

mean and range of
upper and lower
95% - confidence interval
as percentage of
potency
(N =28)

number of animals per dilution

RIVM 20793

Fig. 2:
95% Confidence interval as a function of the size of the groups
of mice used per vaccine dilution in the potency assay on the
diphtheria component in vaccines.

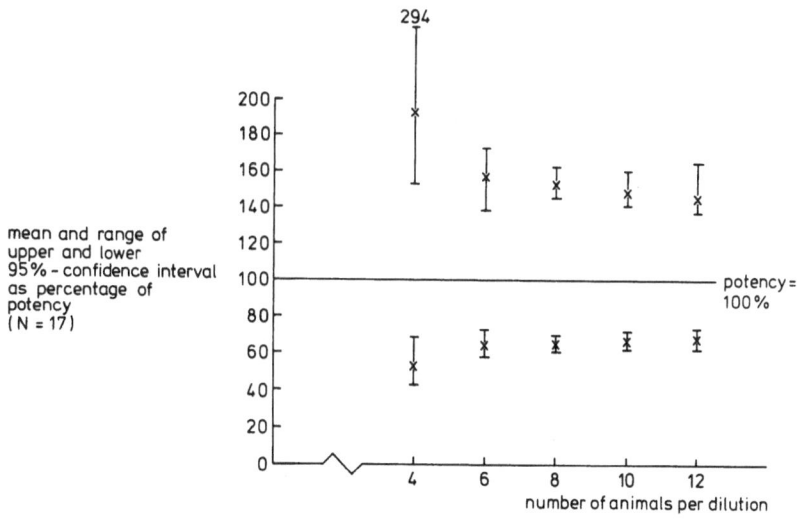

mean and range of
upper and lower
95% - confidence interval
as percentage of
potency
(N = 17)

number of animals per dilution

RIVM 20795

Alternative 3 is the best choice from an ethical, economic (the cost of the mouse model is only one fiftieth of that of the traditional potency assay in guina pigs (33)) and scientific point of view. This method has already been adopted by the Dutch control authorities, which means that some 2400 animals can be spared annually.

It should be emphasized, however, that the number of animals required for whatever method can only be reduced if both vaccine production and control are consistent, as is indeed the case with many manufacturers of human vaccines. Furthermore, comprehensive potency testing will still be necessary whenever a high degree of precision is required such as in the calibration of the reference preparations.

Finally, three other approaches can be mentioned which may lead to a further reduction or refinement of animal usage in the potency testing of diphtheria and, possibly, other vaccines. These are:

1) Reducing the number of vaccine dilutions: 1 dilution of the reference vaccine and 1 dilution of the product under examination. This is the so-called two-point assay which is based on the principle that the test vaccine can be regarded as an unknown dilution of the reference preparation (the parallel-line bioassay concept). A clear understanding of the variations in the dose-response curves of the two types of preparation is important here. It is therefore essential to have a thoroughly validated and consistent production process.

2) Discontinuing the routine use of a standard preparation in each assay. The purpose of a standard preparation is to minimize the influence of such variables as housing, diet, genetic material and the like, on the outcome of the test. However, many of these variables are now standardized, partly owing to the implementation of the Code of Good Laboratory Practice (GLP). From this angle, it is advisable to examine how great the influence of these variables is on the current test, that is, how great is the intervariability of the different assays. When this is smaller than the intravariability within one and the same assay (caused, among other things, by the individual sensitivity of the animals), then there is no longer any need for including a standard preparation in each new test, and the data on the standard preparation obtained from, for example, a half-yearly check will be sufficient.

3) Developing an in vitro model. In this connection, basic research has been carried out on the so-called lymphocyte stimulation model (35, 36), in which sensitized (human) B and T lymphocytes are brought into culture. The addition of antigen stimulates the B-lymphocytes to produce antibodies, a process which is both antigen-dose dependent and antigen specific. Further study showed that the amount of (neutralizing) antibody can be estimated by in vitro neutralization in Vero cells. Therefore, the combination of in vitro lymphocyte stimulation and in vitro neutralization appears to be a suitable functional parameter for estimating the potency of a vaccine product entirely in vitro. However, several problems will have to be solved before this in vitro potency assay can be used for routine use, but this model looks promising enough to merit further research.

The quantitative 3+3 bioassay for determining the potency of the diphtheria component of vaccines is still the most commonly used

assay throughout the world, both for routine batch testing and
for calibration of standard preparations. As was shown above, if
production satisfies the condition of consistency then the
accurate estimation of the potency for routine control can be
regarded as superfluous. For a reduction and refinement of the
use of animals, several approaches can be followed, including
both quantitative and qualitative methods. Thus, with certain
determinations, such as the calibration of standard preparations,
an accurate, and thus quantitative, test is still required. The
serum neutralization test could be used for this purpose, with
the possibility of combining it with _in vitro_ stimulation of
human lymphocytes in the future. However, for the routine testing
of vaccines a qualitative test, such as the "two-point" assay,
may in certain circumstances be sufficient.

4.4. <u>Abnormal toxicity test</u>
See section 2.3.

5. PERTUSSIS VACCINE

The whooping cough, or pertussis vaccine, consists of a
suspension of Bordetella pertussis killed by heating. It is a
whole-cell product, that is, it contains inactivated but
otherwise intact bacteria. Pertussis vaccine is usually
administered as a triple vaccine, the other two components being
tetanus and diphtheria. Pertussis vaccine is one of the most
troublesome vaccine products. Because of its complex structure as
a whole-cell vaccine, it contains biologically active components
which can provoke adverse reactions in vaccine recipients. The
lymphocytosis promoting factor (LPF) and the endotoxin (a
lipopolysaccharide) can be mentioned in this connection. As a
result, there is a narrow margin between the amount of antigen
needed to induce effective immunity and that giving rise to side
effects. This has led to stringent requirements for the quality
control of this vaccine, which is reflected in the relatively
high number of experimental animals used for this product
anually. To give an impression: of the 250,000 animals needed for
the standardization of biological products in the Netherlands,
21,000 were used in the quality control of the pertussis vaccine.
Animal tests play an important role both during the in-process
control and in the final control.
The following tests are here relevant:
- test for specific toxicity;
- potency test;
- test for endotoxins (not statutory);
- test for abnormal toxicity.

5.1. <u>Specific-toxicity test</u>
Various methods are available for this purpose. The mouse-weight-
gain test and the hyperinsulinaemia/hypoglycaemia test (37)
emerged as the most appropriate models from a comparative study
(38). The aspecific mouse-weight-gain test finds general
application. The principle of this test is based on the effect of
toxic vaccine components on the weight gain of growing mice. The
vaccine is administered intraperitoneally to a group of animals.
Its efficacy is assessed from the change in weight between the
first and the seventh (last) day of the experiment. It was shown
that various factors such as mouse strain, diet, etc., can
influence the outcome of the test so that a control group must
also be included (39).

To evaluate the test results, the growth curve of the vaccinated
mice is related to that of the control group.
Table 11 summarizes the guidelines and their specifications for
the mouse-weight-gain test.

Table 11: SPECIFICATIONS OF THE GUIDELINES FOR THE MOUSE-
WEIGHT-GAIN TEST

Specifications	Distress category 1*				
	WHO (40)	Eur.Ph. (2)	Neth. (3)	USA (5)	Japan (6)
Species	mouse	n.s.	mouse	mouse	mouse
No. of animal groups	1		1	1	n.s.
No. of animals/group	≥10		12	10	10
No. of control groups	1		1	no	yes,n.s.
- no. of animals/group	≥10		12		10
Route of administration	i.p.		i.p.	i.p.	i.p.
Observation period (days)	7		7	7	7
Criterion	.... weight				

*   See chapter 5, section 4
n.s. = not specified;   i.p. = intraperitoneal.

This table shows that the number of animals specified by the
various guidelines for this test differs. The Dutch requirement
of 20 mice per group is rather high, and a reduction to 10 to 15
animals might be acceptable. However, the possible toxicity of
the pertussis vaccine demands a cautious policy. The requirement
for a control group has already been mentioned. It could be
useful to look into the possibility of constructing a mean growth
curve for the mouse strain used from the existing data, and to
use this reference in the test instead of a control group.
However, it should be realized that the resulting saving on the
number of animals achievable can never be fully utilized,since
any deviation from the normal course of a test without a control
group will certainly lead to the test being repeated.

5.2. Potency test
Examination for this aspect - which occurs during both the in-
process control and the final control - is based universally on
the intracerebral (lethal) challenge test. Groups of mice are
injected with virulent Bordetella pertussis bacteria after a
given immunization period. The criterion by which the results are
evaluated is death. A correlation with the protective activity in
man has been demonstrated in field trials (41). Table 12 lists
the existing guidelines and their specifications for this test.
Although the experiment causes appreciable pain to the animals
and has its shortcomings, no opportunities for replacement or
refinement are currently available. Because of the narrow margin
between the effective and the toxic dose of this vaccine, a
statistically reliable assay is essential, ruling out a reduction
in the size of the groups, or the introduction of a qualitative
assay. The numbers mentioned in the guidelines, 16 animals per
dilution, are mostly theoretical, and larger numbers are
generally used in practice.

Table 12: SPECIFICATIONS OF THE EXISTING GUIDELINES FOR THE
POTENCY ASSAY ON THE PERTUSSIS VACCINE

Specifications	WHO (40)	Eur.Ph. (2)	Neth. (3)	UK (4)	USA (5)	Japan (6)
Species	mouse	mouse	mouse	mouse	mouse	mouse
No. of animal groups	3	3	3	3	3	3
No. of animals/group	≥16	≥16	20	16	≥16	≥16
Route of administration	i.p.	i.p.	i.p.	i.p.	i.p.	i.p.
Duration:						
- immunization (days)	14	14-17	14	10-14	14-17	21
- assessment after challenge (days)	14	14	14	14	14	14
No. of control groups	4	4	4	4	4	3
- no. of animals/group	12	10	12	10	≥10	≥10
Reference vaccine	yes	yes	yes	yes	yes	yes
- no. of animal groups	3	3	3	3	3	3
- no. of animals/group	≥16	≥16	20	16	≥16	≥16
Mode of challenge	i.c.	i.c.	i.c.	i.c.	i.c.	i.c.
Criterion	.... death					

*   See chapter 5, section 4
i.c. = intracerebral;   i.p. = intraperitoneal.

5.3. Test for endotoxins
This test is not statutory. See Section 3.3. of this chapter.

5.4. Test for abnormal toxicity
See Section 2.3. of this chapter.

5.5. Future
There is little prospect of reducing or refining the use of
animals in the quality control of the current whole-cell
pertussis vaccine. However, there are developments in the field
of pertussis vaccine production which could have far-reaching
consequences for animal experimentation. The Sato (purified
pertussis) vaccine (42) has recently been investigated in a field
trial in Sweden (43). This is an acellular subunit vaccine
consisting of two immunogenic components of Bordetella pertussis,
namely, detoxified lymphocytosis promoting factor (LPF) and
filamentous haemagglutinin (FHA). Work on such an acellular
product is also in progress at other centres around the world. To
all appearances the whole-cell vaccine will be replaced by an
acellular product within a few years.
It is generally believed that neither the intracerebral challenge
nor the mouse-weight-gain test will be satisfactory models for
the control of the acellular vaccine (44). Since the acellular
product induces a better defined immunity than the whole-cell
vaccine, it may be possible to estimate its potency by serum
neutralization using Chinese hamster ovary (CHO) cells (45) or by
an ELISA assay. Both methods have recently been validated and
will, if included in the requirements, lead to a reduction and
refinement of the use of laboratory animals.

6. TETANUS VACCINE

The diphtheria and tetanus vaccines belong to the same category
because both contain a toxoid as the immunogenic component. The
toxoid of the tetanus vaccine is obtained by detoxifying the
toxin of Clostridium tetani bacteria with formaldehyde. The
tetanus toxoid is included in the National Vaccination Programme
in the Netherlands. The following quality control tests are
relevant to the objectives - the 3 Rs - of this project:
- identity test;
- test for specific toxicity;
- potency test;
- test for abnormal toxicity.

6.1. Identity test
There are both _in vivo_ and _in vitro_ methods available for the
identity test. The _in vitro_ methods are usually the same as those
used in the identity test of the diphtheria vaccine (section
4.1.). The Dutch guidelines stipulate an _in vitro_ assay (the
flocculation test).

6.2. Test for specific toxicity
If vaccine contains free toxin, which may occur as a result of
incomplete inactivation, vaccination gives rise to severe side
effects. The purpose of testing for specific toxicity is to
prevent such complications. Groups of guinea pigs are injected
subcutaneously with an excess of the vaccine product, followed by
an observation period of 4 to 6 weeks. The presence of free toxin
leads to symptoms of tetanus. The test is performed both during
the in-process control on the unpurified product and in the final
control on the purified toxoid and the adsorbed vaccine. Table 13
summarizes the existing guidelines and their specifications for
the final control test.

Table 13: SPECIFICATIONS OF THE EXISTING GUIDELINES FOR THE
          SPECIFIC-TOXICITY TEST ON THE TETANUS VACCINE

	Distress category 1 - 4*				
Specifications	WHO (1)	Eur.Ph. (46)	Neth. (3)	UK (4)	Japan (6)
Species	guinea pig	guinea pig	guinea pig	guinea pig	guinea pig
No. of animal groups	1	1	1	1	1
No. of animals/group	5	5	5	5	4
Route of administration	s.c.	s.c.	s.c.	s.c.	s.c.
Observation period (days)	21	30	21	30	21
Criterion	.... tetanus signs				

*   See chapter 5, section 4
s.c. = subcutaneous

There is agreement on the mode of administration and the
criterion used to evaluate the outcome, while small differences
exist as regards the number of animals to be used and the length
of the observation period.

A slight reduction in the number of animals can be achieved by bringing the specifications into line with those of the Japanese guidelines. A further reduction is not possible, but an effort should be made to minimize the frequency of this test during the in-process batch control for the same reason as was given at the discussion of the diphtheria vaccine (see section 4.2.). The test can be refined by killing all animals showing the first signs of tetanus intoxication, i.e., a characteristic gait and spastic paralysis of the hind legs.

The use of gangliosides, the nerve cell binding sites for tetanus toxin, as an alternative to the in vivo test for specific toxicity has been investigated (unpublished observations). This study was based on data from the literature indicating that tetanus toxoid (i.e., the completely detoxified toxin), unlike the toxin, can no longer bind to gangliosides (53). However, experiments with ganglioside-coated ELISA plates showed that there is some binding when the toxoid is present in high concentrations, so that this model is unsuitable for the detection of incompletely detoxified toxin.

6.3. Potency test

The remarks made concerning the opportunities for in vitro techniques, such as haemagglutination and ELISA, in the potency testing of the diphtheria vaccine (section 4.3.) This test is as yet entirely based on in vivo methods.

Table 14 lists the guidelines and their specifications for this test.

As with the potency test for the diphtheria vaccine, a striking feature is here too the marked difference between the US guidelines' requirements and those of the other countries. For a discussion of this difference the reader is referred to section 4.3. of this chapter.

The guidelines are in broad agreement as regards the mode of administration and challenge, the use of a reference preparation and the number of animals to be used (the WHO guidelines give no specifications; the only condition made is that enough animals should be included to make the 95% confidence interval fall within the range of 50-200% of the potency).

The guidelines differ as to the number of control groups and to the number of control animals required to determine the LD50 of the challenging toxin and the assessment criterion to be used. The number of control animals needed for this LD50 determination can be reduced by bringing the specifications into line with those of the WHO.

It is more difficult to make a recommendation on the assessment criterion to be used. On the one hand, using paralysis as the criterion constitutes a refinement in comparison with the traditional challenge (lethality) by reducing considerably the distress caused (47) but, on the other hand, paralysis is sometimes difficult to diagnose so that the assessment of the clinical picture becomes a subjective criterion. As a result, the test has to be repeated in some cases.

The choice between paralytic challenge and lethal challenge is consequently a weighing-up of pros and cons for which no compulsory rules can be prescribed.

However, the lethal challenge can be refined by killing the animals as soon as unambiguous signs of tetanus develop.

Table 14: SPECIFICATIONS OF THE EXISTING GUIDELINES FOR THE
POTENCY TEST ON THE TETANUS VACCINE

Specifications	Distress category 4*					
	WHO (1)	Eur.Ph. (52)	Neth. (3)	UK (4)	USA** (22)	Japan*** (6)
Species	guinea pig/ mouse	guinea pig/ mouse	mouse	guinea pig/ mouse	guinea pig	guinea pig
No. of animal groups	3	3	3	3	1	n.s.
No. of animals/group	n.s.	16	20	16	4	≥10
Route of administration	s.c	s.c.	s.c.	s.c.	n.s.	s.c.
Duration:						
- immunization (days)	28	28	21	28	n.s.	28-42
- assessment after challenge (days)	5	5	5	5		7
No. of control groups	3	4	1	4	1	3
- no. of animals/group	2/4	5/6	10	5/6	2	n.s.
Reference vaccine	yes	yes	yes	yes	no	yes
- no. of animal groups	3	3	3	3	-	n.s.
- no. of animals/group	n.s.	16	20	16	-	n.s.
Mode of challenge	s.c.	s.c.	s.c.	s.c.	-	n.s.
Criterion	d/p	d/p	d	p	titration in 6 mice	d

*	See chapter 5, section 4
**	US requirements for adsorbed tetanus toxoid
***	The Japanese guidelines state that the antitoxin titration method may be used as an alternative to the in vivo lethal challenge test.

n.s. = not specified;   s.c. = subcutaneous
d   = death   p   = paralysis

6.3.1. Reduction of group size

As for the potency testing of the diphtheria vaccine, the author
similarly made a computer study of the possibilities of reducing
the number of animals for the potency assay (29). The individual
data on the animals were known for seven tetanus vaccine batches.
Of these 7 vaccine batches, the potency of which had previously
been established by the traditional lethal challenge test with 20
animals per group, the potency and its 95% confidence interval
were recalculated on the basis of hypothetically composed animal
groups.
Table 15 summarizes the values obtained for group sizes of 20,
16, 14, 12, 10 and 8 animals per vaccine dilution. Some of the
re-examined vaccine batches were for veterinary use, for which
the European Pharmacopoeia gives no minimum requirements.
Figure 3 shows the effect of group size on the 95% confidence
interval. It can be deduced that 60% of the number of animals
currently required [20] would have been sufficient for estimating
the vaccine's potency within the limits of the 95% confidence
interval set by the WHO. This means a potential saving of about
2000 mice per year in the Netherlands. The fact that two research
groups in Britain and Canada arrived at the same conclusion
increases the importance of this statement. On the basis of these
findings an informal working party formulated several proposals
for the potency testing of the tetanus (and the diphtheria)

Table 15: THE EFFECT OF A REDUCTION IN THE NUMBERS OF ANIMALS ON
THE ESTIMATE OF POTENCY AND THE 95% CONFIDENCE INTERVAL
FOR 7 BATCHES OF VACCINE IN THE TETANUS LETHAL
CHALLENGE TEST

	Number of mice per dilution and potency in IU/ml										
	20		16		14		12		10		8	
Batch number	IU/ml	95% interval	IU/ml	95% interval	IU/ml	95% interval	IU/ml	95% interval	IU/ml	95% interval	IU/ml	95% interval
W	119	83-171	122	81-184	110	73-167	118	73-191	95	59-151	91	51-161
X	209	146-295	213	140-317	201	109-331	226	114-397	204	77-410	209	105-389
T77A10	279	195-399	257	168-390	235	153-352	266	163-420	253	139-435	257	132-485
T80	209	142-308	222	139-354	134	140-393	205	119-349	183	94-345	141	62-283
DPT-polio 136*	131	91-188	113	72-174	127	80-203	130	78-213	144	79-260	128	63-246
Y	259	179-400	251	169-399	214	141-341	235	150-391	248	153-428	235	135-446
Z	220	151-335	205	135-324	208	135-334	213	133-357	191	117-324	186	107-345

* D=Diphtheria,   P=Pertussis,   T=Tetanus
  IU=International Units
W, X, Y and Z are batches for veterinary application

component in vaccines (33), and submitted these to the WHO in December 1985. The essence of these proposals was that a considerable reduction in the number of animals used per vaccine dilution is feasible, based on a confidence interval of 50-200% of the potency and a demonstrated consistency in production and control. They have recently been adopted by the WHO (34).
A differentiated approach to potency testing is required to enable a further replacement, reduction or refinement of animal usage, and is linked to the possibilities that exist for the potency test on the diphtheria vaccine, namely:
- reduction of the number of vaccine dilutions;
- discontinuation of the use of the standard vaccine in each test;
- development of an in vitro model based on lymphocyte stimulation;
- in vitro determination of the antibody titre.
The reader is referred to section 4.3.3. for a detailed discussion of this subject. The development of an in vitro model holds good prospects. Preliminary results of recent studies (48) give rise to optimism. These studies indicated that tetanus toxoid can induce human peripheral blood lymphocytes to synthesize specific antibodies in a dose-dependent manner. This model will be validated shortly. Meanwhile, the possibility of estimating the amount of neutralizing antibodies (produced in vivo or in vitro) will have to be examined. There are several references to a specific ELISA assay, based on microtitre plates coated with purified tetanus toxoid. However, a limitation of this direct determination of the tetanus antibody titre is that the method does not discriminate between neutralizing (protective) and non-neutralizing (non-protective) antibodies. As a result, there exists a poor correlation between the Toxoid-ELISA assay and the in vivo assay. Recently an in vitro method was described (54) by which the tetanus antibody titre can be estimated in human sera. It is based on the determination of free tetanus toxin by an ELISA following pre-incubation of serum dilutions with constant amounts of toxin. This method gives a good correlation with the in vivo assay. The usefulness of this approach for estimating the potency of tetanus toxoid is currently under investigation.

6.4. Test for abnormal toxicity
See section 2.3. of this chapter.

7. TYPHOID VACCINE

The starting material for this vaccine is an inactivated culture of Salmonella typhi bacteria. These bacteria must contain antigens of types O, H and Vi. As regards the objectives of this project, the following tests are relevant to the quality control of the typhoid vaccine (which has a limited production volume):
- test for endotoxins;
- potency test;
- test for abnormal toxicity.

Figure 3:
Mean and range of upper and lower 95% confidence interval as
percentage of potency (N=7)

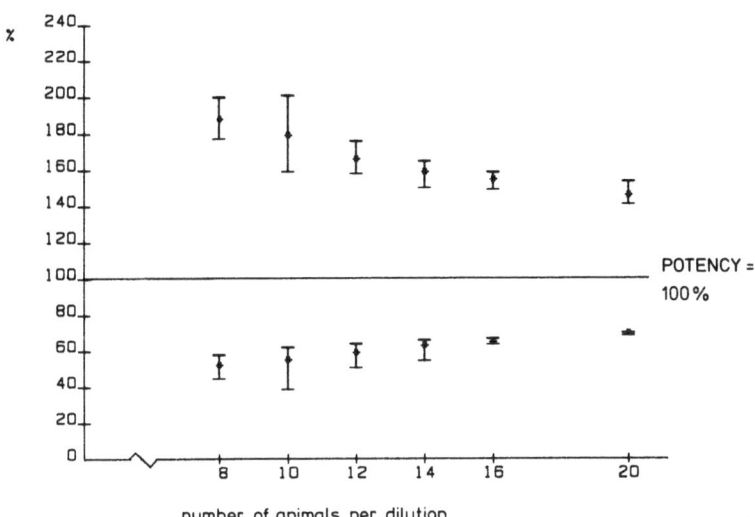

number of animals per dilution

7.1. <u>Test for endotoxins</u>
See section 3.3. of this chapter.

7.2. <u>Potency test</u>
Table 16 summarizes the existing guidelines and their
specifications for this test.
Although field trials indicated that the typhoid vaccine has
moderate protective activity (50), there is as yet little insight
into the nature of the immunity induced by it. This is partly
related to the fact that no suitable animal model is available
for research on the typhoid vaccine or for testing its efficacy.

Table 16: SPECIFICATIONS OF THE VARIOUS GUIDELINES FOR THE
POTENCY TEST ON TYPHOID VACCINE

Specifications	WHO (49)	Eur.Ph. (2)	Distress category 2* Neth. (3)	USA (5)	Japan (6)
Species	mouse/ rabbit	n.s.	rabbit	mouse	guinea pig
No. of animal groups	n.s.	n.s.	1	≥ 3	1
No. of animals/group	n.s.	n.s.	3	≥16	≥ 8
Route of administration	n.s.	n.s.	i.v.	i.p.	i.p.
Duration:					
- immunization (days)	n.s.	n.s.	15	7-14	14
- assessment after challenge (days)			-	3	14
No. of control groups			no	≥ 4	1
- no. of animals/group				≥10	≥ 8
Reference vaccine	n.s.	n.s.	no	yes	no
Mode of challenge				i.p.	i.p.
Criterion	c/a	a	a	c	c

```
*       See chapter 5, section 4
n.s. = not specified;            i.v. = intravenous;
i.p. = intraperitoneal;          c    = challenge;
a    = antibodies to O, H and Vi;
```

It is true that mice can be protected against artificial typhoid
infection by vaccination, but the results of these experiments do
not show satisfactory correlation with the results of
immunization trials in man (51). Any potency assay based on a
mouse model is therefore not very relevant. Without suggesting by
this that a serological test in rabbits is a better model, it is
nevertheless preferable to the mouse model from an animal-ethical
point of view (no lethal challenge, fewer animals).

7.3. Test for abnormal/specific toxicity
The Dutch guidelines specify a combined test for abnormal and
specific toxicity. It is based on 3 guinea pigs and 10 mice, but
is otherwise the same as the test for abnormal toxicity, that is,
the weight of the animals is used as the assesment criterion.
(Note: specific clinical symptoms of typhoid do not develop in
mice and guinea pigs). No proposals to reduce or refine this test
can be made from the available data.

8. SUMMARY

As far as is possible to survey, the following approaches towards
reduction or refinement of animal usage in the quality control of
human vaccines can be, or already have been, implemented.

In the short term (within 5 years)
- GENERAL:
    - reduction of the numbers of animals used for testing for
      abnormal toxicity;
    - reduction of the frequency of the abnormal toxicity test by
      increasing the capacity of the packaging equipment;
    - application of the LAL test for detecting the presence of
      endotoxins (the test is not mandatory).

- DIPHTHERIA VACCINE
  - specific toxicity: - decreased frequency of this test;
                       - replacement of the guinea pig model by a
                         tissue culture method (Vero cells).
  - potency: - replacement of the lethal challenge by
                         serum neutralization in tissue culture
                         (based on the mouse model with a limited
                         number of animals); this has already
                         been introduced in the Netherlands;
                         estimated saving was around 2400 animals
                         in 1986;
                       - possible reduction of the number of
                         vaccine dilutions and/or omission of
                         thereference vaccine.

- PERTUSSIS VACCINE
  - specific toxicity: - possible omission of the control group.

- TETANUS VACCINE
  - potency: - reduction of the number of animals
                         required per vaccine dilution (to around
                         12); this has already been implemented
                         in the Netherlands; estimated saving was
                         around 2000 animals in 1986;
                       - possible reduction of the number of
                         vaccine dilutions and/or omission of the
                         reference vaccine.
  - specific toxicity: - decreased frequency of this test.

In the medium term (5-10 years)
- PERTUSSIS VACCINE (based on the subunit vaccine if it proves
  effective)
  - potency: - replacement of the lethal
                         intracerebralchallenge procedure in mice
                         with a serum antibody assay in tissue
                         culture (serum neutralization) or by an
                         ELISA assay.
  - specific toxicity: - replacement of the guinea pig model by
                         an assay in tissue culture (an in vitro
                         determination in microtitre plates
                         coated with gangliosides).
- TETANUS VACCINE
  - potency: - replacement of the lethal challenge by
                         toxin binding inhibition test in ELISA
                         plates

Realization of the above-mentioned alternative approaches to the
potency testing of the tetanus and pertussis vaccines opens the
possibility to combine the potency assay of the pertussis, the
tetanus and the diphtheria vaccine into one experiment. This
would greately decrease the total number of animals used.

- GENERAL
  - Potency: - replacement of the in vivo by in vitro
                         models, for example, based on lymphocyte
                         stimulation. Validation studies need to
                         be carried out for both the diphtheria
                         and the tetanus components in vaccines.
                         The potency assay for the pertussis
                         vaccine still requires basic research.

90

9. REFERENCES

1. WHO, Technical Report Series 638 (1979).
2. European Pharmacopoeia, Mon. 163 (1984).
3. Werkvoorschriften Laboratorium Controle Bacteriële Vaccins. (Methods for testing of bacterial vaccines.) RIVM, The Netherlands.
4. British Pharmacopoeia, Vol. II, (1980).
5. Code of Federal Regulations, FDA, No. 21, 600-799, (1982).
6. Minimum requirements of biological products, (1982), Ministry of Health and Welfare, Japanese Government.
7. WHO, Technical Report Series 413, (1969).
8. European Pharmacopoeia, Vol. II, (1971).
9. Round Table Conference: safety tests on veterinary products and abnormal-toxicity tests on products in human medicine, Symposium IABS, April 1985, London. Develop. Biol. Standard. (1986), 64, 309.
10. Booth, C.: The limulus amoebocyte lysate (LAL) assay - Areplacement for the rabbit pyrogen test. Develop. Biol. Standard. (1986), 64, 271-275.
11. Levin, J. and Bang, F.B.: The role of endotoxin in the extracellular coagulation of limulus blood. Bull. Johns Hopkins Hosp. (1964), 115, 265.
12. Cooper, J.F. et al.: The limulus test for endotoxin (pyrogen)in radiopharmaceuticals and biologicals. Bull. Parenteral Drug Assoc. (1972), 26, 153-162.
13. Kreeftenberg, J.G. et al.: The limulus amebocyte lysate test micromethod and application in the control of sera and vaccines. Develop. Biol. Standard. (1977), 34, 15-20.
14. Sullivan, J.D. and Watson, S.W.: Factors affecting the sensitivity of limulus lysate. Appl. Microbiol. (1974), 28, 1023-26.
15. European Pharmacopoeia, Mon. 154 (1982).
16. Oseasohn, R.O. et al.: Field trial of cholera vaccine in rural East Pakistan. The Lancet (1965), Febr. 27, 450-452.
17. Guinee, P.A.M. et al.: Vibrio cholera infection and acquiredimmunity in an adult rabbit model. Zbl. Bakt. Hyg, (1984), A259, 118-131.
18. Winsnes, R. and Mogster, B.: The identification of diphtheria, tetanus and pertussis vaccines by single radial and double immunodiffusion techniques. Journ. Biol. Standard. (1985), 13, 31-34.
19. European Pharmacopoeia, Mon. 443 (1985).
20. Abrea, C.B. and Stainer, D.W.: A tissue culture assay for diphtheria toxicity testing. Develop.Biol.Standard (1986), 64, 33-37.
21. Gun, J. van der: Personal communication.
22. Hardegree, M.C.: WHO ad hoc meeting: potency testing of toxoids. Geneva, December 12-14, 1983.
23. Stainer, D.W. and Hart, F.E.: The development of reliable and economic methods for the assay of tetanus and diphteria toxoids. WHO ad hoc meeting, Geneva, December 12-14, 1983.
24. Anonymus: Report on an informal consultation on the potency assay of diphtheria and tetanus toxoids. WHO ad hoc meeting, Geneva, December 12-14, 1983.
25. Knight, P.A.: The evaluation of the response of guinea pigs to diphtheria toxoids. Journ. Biol. Standard. (1974), 2, 69-78.

26. Kreeftenberg, J.G. et al.: An investigation of a mouse model to estimate the potency of the diphtheria component in vaccines. Journ. Biol. Standard. (1985), 13, 229-234.
27. Kreeftenberg. J.G. et al.: A mouse model to estimate the potency of the diphtheria component in combined vaccines. Develop. Biol. Standard. (1986), 64, 21-24.
28. Miyamura, K. et al.: Micro-cell culture method for determination of diphtheria toxin and antitoxin titres using VERO-cells. Journ. Biol. Standard. (1974), 2, 203-209.
29. Hendriksen, C.F.M. et al.: The effects of reductions in the numbers of animals used for the potency assay of the diphtheria and tetanus components of adsorbed vaccines by the methods of the European Pharmacopoeia. Jour. Biol. Standard. (1987), 15, 353-362.
30. Knight, P.A. and Roberts, P.A.G.: Studies on the minimal number of animals required to achieve assurance of satisfactory potency in diphtheria and tetanus vaccines. 19th IABS Congress on Use and Standardization of Combined Vaccines, Amsterdam, the Netherlands, 1985. Develop. Biol. Standard. (1986), 65.
31. Knight, P.A. and Roberts, P.A.G.: An evaluation of some proposals for a reduction in the number of animals used for the potency testing of diphtheria and tetanus vaccines. Jour. Biol. Standard. (1987), 15, 165-177.
32. Stainer, D.W. et al.: Reduction in animal usage for potency testing of diphtheria and tetanus toxoids. 19th IABS Congress on Use and Standardization of Combined Vaccines, Amsterdam, the Netherlands, 1985. Develop. Biol. Standard. (1986), 65, 241-244.
33. Kreeftenberg, J.G.: Informal meeting about alternative methods for the potency control of diphtheria and tetanus components in vaccines. 19th IABS Congress on Use and Standardization of Combined Vaccines, Amsterdam, the Netherlands, 1985. Develop. Biol. Standard. (1986), 65, 261-267.
34. WHO, Technical Report Series 760 (1987).
35. Kreeftenberg, J.G. et al.: Investigations on the immunogenicity of tetanus vaccine in vitro. Sixth International Conference on Tetanus. December 3-5, 1981. Lyon. Fondation Marcel Mérieux.
36. Uyt de Haag, F.G.C.M. et al.: Induction of antigen-specific antibody response in human peripheral blood lymphocytes in vitro by a dog kidney cell vaccine against rabies virus (DKCV). The Journal of Immunology, (1983), 131, 3, 1234-39.
37. Kreeftenberg, J.G. et al.: A biphasic serum glucose responsein mice to inoculation with pertussis vaccine. Journ. Biol. Standard. (1984), 12, 151-157.
38. Hooker, J.M.: A laboratory study of the toxicity of some diphtheria-tetanus-pertussis vaccines. Journ. Biol. Standard. (1981), 9, 493-506.
39. Pittman, M. and Cox, B.: Pertussis vaccine testing for freedom-from-toxicity. Appl. Microbiol. (1965), 13, 3, 447-456.
40. WHO Document, BLG/UNDP/82.1. Rev 1, 1982.
41. Medical Research Council: Vaccination against whooping cough:relation between protection in children and results of laboratory tests. Brit. Med. J., (1956), 2, 454.
42. Sato, Y. et al.: Development of a pertussis component vaccine in Japan. The Lancet, (1984), Jan. 21, 122-126.

43. Granström, M. et al.: Antitoxin response to acellular
    pertussis vaccine. Annual Meeting Am. Soc. Micr., Wash. D.C.
    (1987), 113.
44. Anonymous: Developments in pertussis vaccines. Memorandum
    from a WHO meeting. Bull. Wld. Hlth. Org. (1985), 63, 2, 241-
    248.
45. Gillenius, P. et al.: The standardization of an assay for
    pertussis toxin and antitoxin in microplate culture of
    Chinese hamster ovary cells. Journ. Biol. Standard. (1985),
    13, 61-66.
46. European Pharmacopoeia, Mon. 452 (1985).
47. Mussett, M.V. and Sheffield, F.: A collaborative
    investigation of a potency assay for adsorbed tetanus
    vaccines based on the protection of mice from tetanic
    paralysis. Journ. Biol. Standard. (1976), 4, 141-148.
48. Loggen, H.G.: Personal communication.
49. WHO Technical Report Series 361 (1967).
50. Yugoslav Typhoid Commission: A controlled field trial of the
    effectiveness of acetone-dried inactivated and heat-phenol
    inactivated typhoid vaccines in Yugoslavia. Bull. Wld. Hlth.
    Org. (1964), 30, 623-630.
51. Cohen, H.: Buiktyfus (Typhoid fever), in: Immunization
    against infectious diseases by F. Dekking et al., published
    in the series entitled Nederlandse Bibliotheek der
    Geneeskunde (Dutch Medical Library) by Stafleu's
    Wetenschappelijke Uitgeversmaatschappij B.V. (1974).
52. European Pharmacopoeia, Mon. 452 (1985).
53. Haberman, E. and Dreyer, F.: Clostridial neurotoxins:
    Handling and action at the cellular and molecular level.
    Current Topics in Microbiology and Immunology (1986), 129,
    93-197.
54. Hendriksen, C.F.M. et al: The toxin binding inhibition test
    as a reliable in vitro alternative to the toxin
    neutralization test in mice for the estimation of tetanus
    antitoxin in human sera. Journ.Biol.Standard. (1988), 16, 4
    (in press).

1. INTRODUCTION

Seven human viral vaccines are produced in the Netherlands for
routine application, namely: 1. mumps vaccine;
2. hepatitis B vaccine;
3. influenza vaccine;
4. measles vaccine;
5. poliomyelitis
vaccine(inactivated);
6. rabies vaccine;
7. rubella (German measles) vaccine.
Of these products, the polio (inactivated), measles and rubella
vaccines and recently also the mumps vaccine are included in the
National Vaccination Programme.
Two different types of polio vaccine have been developed. Most
countries use the live, attenuated polio vaccine which is
administered orally. The other product is the killed, or
inactivated, polio vaccine. The Netherlands, the Scandinavian
nations and parts of Canada use the latter. Both the live, oral
and the inactivated polio vaccines will be reviewed here.
Compared with the human bacterial vaccines, the number of animals
used for the viral vaccines is relatively low. This is partly
because of the nature of the product, especially of the live
vaccines. A second reason is that in the last few decades there
has already been considerable replacement and reduction of animal
usage in the case of the viral vaccines. The most important
animal tests are those for testing for the presence of extraneous
microorganisms, for potency testing (for the inactivated vaccines
only), and for abnormal-toxicity testing. The following table
shows the production and control aspects for each of the vaccines
as well as the possibilities of using alternative methods.

test for abnormal toxicity	test for extraneous agents	tumourigenicity test	test for residual live virus	potency test	production	
±	-	0	0	0	0	Mumps vaccine
±	±	0	±	-	0	Hepatitis B vaccine
±	0	0	0	+	0	Influenza vaccine
±	-	0	0	0	0	Measles vaccine
±	±	±	+	-	±	Poliomyelitis vaccine (inactivated)
±	+	±	0	0	+	Poliomyelistis vaccine (live oral)
±	±	0	±	±	-	Rabies vaccine
±	-	0	0	0	+	Rubella vaccine

Legend: see chapter 8, table 1 for an explanation of the symbols.

Each vaccine product is discussed in turn in the following sections, and a summary concludes the chapter. However, a few general remarks should first be made about the test for extraneous microorganisms.

2. TESTS FOR EXTRANEOUS MICROORGANISMS

The product must be monitored for microbial contamination during the entire manufacturing process; this applies in particular to the live vaccines, since any undesirable microorganisms will be co-cultured with the vaccine virus. This quality control consists of a number of complementary tests, usually in vitro techniques (serological assays and tissue culture systems) as well as several animal studies. As a rule, the latter consist of two general tests (one in adult and one in newborn mice) and one or more specific tests. The frequency and extent of these animal tests are stongly related to the condition of the animals used for supplying the production cultures. If the cultures are derived from colonies that are free from infectious agents, then the animal test for extraneous microorganisms can be confined to the virus harvest (crude virus suspension, see chapter 4, table 4).
But if conventional animals are used (for example, until recently imported wild-caught monkeys for the polio vaccine) then animal tests must also be performed on the production cells.
The extent of animal testing also depends on the animal species used for the tissue culture. When, for example, rabbits are used (as for the rubella vaccine), then the crude virus suspension is also checked in rabbits in addition to the general animal tests on it, in order to detect species-specific viral contamination. Apart from these tests, which are aimed at viral contamination, tests on laboratory animals may also be performed to detect possible contamination with Mycobacterium tuberculosis and other microorganisms.

3. MUMPS VACCINE

The mumps vaccine produced in the Netherlands for vaccination purposes is a live attenuated, freeze-dried product, grown on cultures of primary chick embryo cells.
The mumps virus has neurotropic properties, and is known to cause neurological complications. Attenuation of the virus for vaccination purposes should therefore eliminate these properties. This is checked whenever a new master seed virus* is put into use, that is, once only.
The master seed virus is tested for neurovirulence by injecting samples of the first five consecutive batches of the new virus vaccine into the brain, spine and muscle of at least 20 monkeys. The replacement of monkeys by smaller laboratory animals is not feasible because the degree of attenuation (and thus the virulence) of the virus strain cannot be established in the latter (2).

---

* This is the stock of seed virus, the "seed lot", which is used for vaccine production for an extended period of time. Some seed virus is taken from this stock for the preparation of each production batch. The master seed virus is stored in liquid nitrogen.

Of the Dutch human vaccines, the mumps vaccine is a relatively
new product. The animal studies performed on this vaccine are
broadly the same as those on the measles vaccine, which will be
described in detail when the latter is discussed (sections 6.1.1.
and 6.1.2.).
The following routine quality control tests are relevant to the
3-R objectives of this project:
- test for extraneous agents (see section 6.1. of this chapter);
- test for abnormal toxicity (see section 2.3. of chapter 8).

4. HEPATITIS B VACCINE

From a production-technical viewpoint, the hepatitis B vaccine
occupies a unique position within the group of viral vaccines.
Unlike most other viruses, the cultivation of the hepatitis B
virus <u>in vitro</u> or in small laboratory animals has so far proved
impossible. However, it is possible to isolate the
immunologically active hepatitis B surface antigen (HBsAG) in
sufficiently large quantities from the plasma of chronic human
carriers, and the currently available hepatitis B vaccines,
including the Dutch one, are based on this. In practice this
means that for vaccine production use is made of selected human
donors.
Since plasma can be a potential source of pathogenic
microorganisms (for example, the AIDS virus) precise requirements
exist for its safety evaluation.
As regards the 3-R objectives of this project, the following
aspects of the routine quality control are important:
- test for extraneous viruses, both in adult and in newborn mice;
- test for freedom from live hepatitis virus;
- potency test;
- test for abnormal toxicity.
For a discussion of the tests for foreign viruses and for
abnormal toxicity the reader is referred to the poliomyelitis
vaccine (section 7.A.3.2. of this chapter) and the BCG vaccine
(chapter 8, section 2.3.) respectively.

4.1. <u>Test for freedom from live hepatitis virus</u>
The hepatitis B vaccine is an inactivated product. Examination of
each newly produced vaccine batch for the absence of live
hepatitis virus forms part of the safety evaluation. To date, the
chimpanzee has been the most suitable animal for this. Two pairs
of animals are injected intravenously with 1 and 10 vaccine doses
respectively, and observed for 6 months. Assessment is made on
the basis of weight, general health, a serological examination,
and a liver biopsy.
The WHO guidelines (3) state that, depending on the results of an
extensive validation of the production process, the test for
residual live virus can either be performed on two animals or be
dispensed with altogether. It is left to the national regulatory
authorities to stipulate how many vaccine batches should be
validated in chimpanzees.

4.2. <u>Potency test</u>
Recommendations for the potency test are made in the Technical
Report Series of the WHO (3). The test is based on a quantitative
assay in mice or guinea pigs, in which groups of at least 20
animals are injected intraperitoneally with various dilutions of
the vaccine under examination or the reference vaccine.

The animals are bled 42 days later and the antibody response is
determined by, e.g., a radioimmunoassay. The efficacy of the new
vaccine product can be calculated from this response.
No methods which could be regarded as alternatives are available
for the potency test. However, a statistical test of the number
of animals required per group is advisable.
A recent development are hepatitis B vaccines produced by
recombinant DNA techniques. The gene coding for HBsAg has been
inserted into yeast or mammalian cells. Studies in mice,
chimpanzees and other species of monkey as well as in humans have
shown that the immunogenicity of these products is similar to
that of the vaccines made from human plasma.
WHO guidelines have been drawn up for the production and quality
control of the recombinant DNA hepatitis B vaccine produced in
yeast. The emphasis is on in-process control. In general, the
tests for potency, pyrogenicity and toxicity are the same as
those for the human plasma-derived vaccine. Because of the
production procedure used, testing for the presence of live
hepatitis virus is no longer necessary.

5. INFLUENZA VACCINE

Inactivated influenza virus vaccine is used for prophylactic
purposes in the Netherlands as well as elsewhere in the world.
The vaccine must contain the most recently isolated strains.
Embryonated hen's eggs are employed for growing the virus.
The influenza vaccine is an encouraging* subject for
consideration in the context of replacement, reduction or
refinement of laboratory animal use, since the animal studies
play only a limited role in its quality control. A few features
of the quality control will be discussed here.

5.1. Potency test
The influenza vaccine is an exception within the group of
inactivated vaccines in that (in most countries) its potency is
not assayed in vivo, although immunogenicity tests based on
animal models do also exist. The in vitro method is based on the
determination of the amount of antigen, the most commonly
technique being single radial immunodiffusion (SRD) (4). It was
already pointed out in previous chapters that the amount of
antigen need not be related to the immunogenic power of the
product. For the influenza vaccine, however, a reasonable
correlation has been found to exist between the amount of antigen
measured with the in vitro potency assay and the protection
conferred in the field.

5.2. Abnormal-toxicity test
See chapter 8, section 2.3.

6. MEASLES VACCINE

A live, attenuated measles virus is used for immunization
purposes in the Netherlands, which is grown on cultures of chick
embryo fibroblasts. This vaccine was included in the National
Vaccination Programme in the Netherlands in 1976.

---

* The author is aware that the use of the word "encouraging", in
  conjunction with the knowledge that chicken embryos are
  required for production purposes, is trivial from a moral
  viewpoint.

Like the mumps virus, the virulent measles virus possesses
neurotropic properties. The attenuated master seed virus is
checked for absence of these properties by the same method as was
described for the mumps vaccine.
The following quality control tests are relevant to the 3-R
objectives of this project:
- test for extraneous agents;
- test for abnormal toxicity.

6.1. Tests for extraneous agents

A distinction can be made between a specific test aimed at
demonstrating the presence of Mycobacterium tuberculosis and two
aspecific tests aimed at foreign viruses.

6.1.1. Test for Mycobacterium tuberculosis

In theory, the cell cultures can be contaminated with avian (via
the donor animal) or with human tuberculosis bacteria (via
laboratory personnel). In practice, however, these sources of
contamination can be excluded because the donor animals are kept
under specific pathogen-free (SPF) conditions, and direct contact
of the personnel with the production cells does not take place,
at least not when the GMP rules are adhered to.
A guinea pig test was until recently stipulated in the
Netherlands for detecting tuberculosis bacteria in the vaccine.
To this end, 5 animals were injected intramuscularly with the
vaccine, and observed for at least 42 days. In most countries,
including the Netherlands, where the above-mentioned hygienic
conditions are satisfied, this in vivo test has been removed from
the quality control, and an in vitro method is used instead.

6.1.2. Test for extraneous viruses

For this test, at least 10 adult mice and at least 20 newborn
mice are injected both intraperitoneally and intracerebrally with
the crude virus suspension, followed by an observation period of
21 and 14 days respectively. The animals should not manifest any
signs of disease during this period. Tables 1 and 2 list the
guidelines and their specifications for this test in adult and
newborn mice respectively.

Table 1: SPECIFICATIONS OF THE EXISTING GUIDELINES FOR THE TEST
FOR EXTRANEOUS VIRUSES IN ADULT MICE

Specifications	Distress category 1*			
	WHO (5)	Neth.(6)	USA (7)	Japan (8)
Species	mouse	mouse	mouse	mouse
No. of animals	≥10	≥10	≥20	≥10
Route of administration	i.p.+i.c.	i.p.+i.c.	i.p.+i.c.	i.p.+i.c.
Control group	no	yes	no	no
- no. of mice		6		
Observation period (days)	21	21	21	21
Criterion	.... Clinical symptoms			
	.... microscopic changes			

* - See chapter 5, section 4
i.p. = intraperitoneal   i.c. = intracerebral

98

Table 2: SPECIFICATIONS OF THE EXISTING GUIDELINES FOR THE TEST
FOR EXTRANEOUS VIRUSES IN NEWBORN MICE

| Specifications | Distress category 1* | | | |
	WHO (5)	Neth.(6)	USA (7)	Japan (8)
Species	mouse	mouse	mouse	mouse
No. of animals	$\geq$20	$\geq$20	$\geq$20	$\geq$20
Route of administration	i.p.+i.c.	i.p.+i.c.	i.p.+i.c.	i.p.+i.c.
Control group	no	yes	no	no
- no. of mice		5		
Observation period (days)	14	14	14	14
Criterion	.... Clinical symptoms			
	.... microscopic changes			

* = See chapter 5, section 4
i.p. = intraperitoneal   i.c. = intracerebral

The various guidelines differ fundamentally as regards the use of
control animals. There are arguments both in favour and against,
and it is difficult to establish which carries most weight. In
favour of a control group is the consideration that, with a
positive finding, a distinction can be made on the basis of the
reaction in the control group between a product-associated cause
and an aspecific cause. However, the fact that aspecific causes
are becoming less and less frequent, which can be ascribed to the
use of high-quality animals and extensive standardization of the
test design, argues against a control group.
Also, regarding the test as a whole, the examination for the
presence of foreign viruses in the measles vaccine (and also in
other viral vaccines) is based on a number of complementary
tests: tissue culture systems, embryonated hen's eggs,
serological assays and in vivo models.
The relevance of the in vivo test may be questioned. Data from 28
laboratories in 16 countries indicated that no foreign viruses
could be demonstrated by animal studies that had not already been
detected in tissue culture (9).
Furthermore, the volume of virus suspension which can be examined
in animals is limited, unlike that in tissue cultures. It is
generally accepted that the number of extraneous particles which
can be detected in a vaccine is related to the volume of the
vaccine sample used (10).
However, none of this is conclusive proof of the irrelevance of
the in vivo models. The reason is that some species of virus
(e.g., lymphocytic choriomeningitis (LCM) virus) can only be
demonstrated in vivo. Moreover, past experience has taught that
in vitro methods cannot always reveal an unknown, sporadically
occurring virus infection. To detect this would require a large
number of tissue culture systems of different cell types. For
these reasons it is not yet feasible to dispense with the animal
test for the detection of extraneous viruses in live vaccines.

6.2. Abnormal-toxicity test
See chapter 8, section 2.3.

7. POLIOMYELITIS VACCINE

There are two types of polio vaccine preparation: the Salk
vaccine, which contains killed polio virus serotypes 1, 2 and 3
and is administered parenterally, and the Sabin vaccine, which
contains live attenuated polio virus (serotypes 1, 2 and 3) and
is given orally. The Netherlands is one of the few countries in
the Western hemisphere where the inactivated product is used. It
was included in 1962 in the National Vaccination Programme. The
two vaccines will be discussed in turn.

7.A. Inactivated poliomyelitis vaccine

The following aspects of the production and control of this
vaccine are relevant to the 3-R objectives of this project:
- production;
- test for residual live virus;
- tests for extraneous agents;
- tumourigenicity test;
- potency test;
- test for abnormal toxicity.

7.A.1. Production

This subject has already been considered in chapter 4. There have
been fundamental changes in the production of the polio virus in
the past few decades. The primary monkey kidney cells, obtained
from monkeys caught in the wild, quarantined for 6-8 weeks and
used initially for growing the virus have gradually been replaced
by subcultured monkey kidney cells from animals born and bred in
captivity. The improved technique not only resulted in a
reduction in the number of animals required but also in a product
of better quality. The developments in polio vaccine production
are thus one of the most striking examples of progress in the
search for alternatives.
However, there are other ways of reducing still further the use
of animals for the production of the polio virus. One way is to
increase the cell harvest per kidney by further refining the
perfusion and trypsinization techniques (11).
Another approach is based on an alternative to the cell substrate
and can - if applied - lead to the complete replacement of the
monkey for production purposes. In this approach, the virus is
cultivated in transformed cells, which are cells capable of
continuous cell division, the so-called continuous cell lines.
These cell lines often possess tumourigenic properties and can
then not be used. The Vero cell line is an exception*, and very
favourable results have been obtained whith this cell line in the
cultivation of the polio virus (12), so it is expected that they
will replace the subcultured cells in the foreseeable future
(13).

7.A.2. Test for residual live virus

In the past, application of the killed polio vaccine (Salk) has
led to several serious accidents which could be attributed to
incomplete inactivation of the vaccine virus. The best known is
the Cutter incident in 1955, named after the American
manufacturer of the vaccine involved. As a result of the use of

---

* Recently, however, tumourigenic properties have been reported
  in Vero cells after they had been passaged many times (14),
  though the number of passages was much higher than is commonly
  used for production purposes.

an incompletely inactivated vaccine batch 250 persons contracted
a poliomyelitis infection of whom five died (1).
Before 1955 testing for residual live virus consisted of a tissue
culture system and an in vivo test in the form of an
intracerebral inoculation in monkeys (Macaca fascicularis). After
1955, the emphasis has been on this monkey test, which was
extended with an intraspinal and intramuscular injection with
virus suspension. However, a recent comparative study (15)
revealed that the tissue culture system is in every respect more
sensitive than the monkey model. In most countries, in accordance
with the WHO requirements, the test in monkeys is now no longer
required, though the United States is an exception to this.
Subcultured monkey kidney cells are used in the in vitro test for
residual live virus (as well as in the test for extraneous
viruses). There are indications that these cells could be
replaced by Vero cells (15), but further research on this is
desirable.

7.A.3. Tests for extraneous agents
As for the measles vaccine, a distinction can here be made
between a specific test aimed at detecting contamination by
Mycobacterium tuberculosis and two aspecific tests for
demonstrating the presence of foreign viruses.

7.A.3.1. Test for Mycobacterium tuberculosis
If monkeys are used from controlled and closed breeding groups
for the production of the polio virus, these animals can be ruled
out as a potential source of contamination provided that the
usually precautionary measures are taken. The same reasoning
therefore applies to the test for the presence of Mycobacterium
tuberculosis in a polio vaccine batch as to the same test on the
measles vaccine (section 6.1.1.).

7.A.3.2. Test for extraneous viruses
The design and execution of the relevant animal studies are the
same as those specified by the guidelines for the measles vaccine
(section 6.1.2, tables 1 and 2). The test in rabbits is aimed
especially at demonstrating the presence of herpesvirus 1 and
other viruses. At least 10 rabbits are injected intradermally and
subcutaneously with the monovalent virus suspension, and
subsequently observed for at least three weeks.
The polio vaccine is an inactivated product. To "guarantee"
complete inactivation, the period required for effective
inactivation of the polio virus is usually exceeded. This has
also consequences for any foreign viruses that may be present.
Only a few virus species are known (e.g. the SV-40 virus) which
resist the inactivation process longer than the poliomyelitis
virus, although the time difference is only small. Consequently,
performing animal tests when sensitive in vitro models for
detecting extraneous viruses are available is debatable. It is
advisable to examine how meaningful in vivo models are for the
test for foreign viruses in inactivated vaccines. The removal of
these tests from the quality control appears feasible.

7.A.4. Tumourigenicity test
There is an increasing tendency to change over to serially
cultivated cells, continuous cell lines (e.g. Vero cells) and
cell strains (e.g. diploid cells) for the production of virus
vaccines. This has focused attention on the possible risk of
transmitting oncogenic material from these cells to vaccinees.

For these cells to be acceptable for production purposes, one of
the current criteria (laid down by the WHO (9) and others) is
therefore the absence of tumourigenic properties. The WHO has two
criteria for tumourigenicity: (a) the development of palpable
nodules increasing in diameter during the observation period of
21 days, and (b) the development of metastases (9).
There are several animal models available for this test, based on
the same principle: two groups of immunosuppressed animals
(athymic mice, newborn hamsters treated with antithymocyte serum,
thymectomized mice, or newborn rats treated with antithymocyte
globulin (ATG) are inoculated with production cells and
neoplastic cells (e.g. HeLa cells) respectively. After an
observation period of 21 days the animals are examined
macroscopically and histologically for the presence of nodules at
the site of injection and for metastases. Nodules should be
present in the control group (injected with HeLa cells), but
absent in the animals injected with the cells intended for
production.
As metastasis occurs in the ATG-treated newborn rat and not in
the other animal models, it seems to be the most suitable for the
in vivo testing of cell substrates for tumourigenicity (16, 17).
Still, the in vivo models exhibit low sensitivity to tumour
formation (17) and in vitro systems are being sought which can be
standardized well, possibly for preliminary screening.
Several alternative approaches have been described, including
organ cultures of chick embryonic skin (18), human muscle
cultures (19) and colony formation in soft agarose (19). A good
correlation has been shown to exist between the test in organ
cultures of chick embryonic skin and various animal tests, but
the former does not provide information about the cells acquiring
invasive growth properties. On the other hand, this capacity can
be observed in the muscle cell culture system.
It may be worthwhile to validate a combination of in vitro models
as a pre-screening test for tumourigenicity testing.

7.A.5. Potency test
Both in vitro (antigenicity) and in vivo (immunogenicity) assays
are available for determining the potency of the killed polio
vaccine. The former category includes a gel immunodiffusion test
(the D-antigen test), a complement fixation test, a
radioimmunoassay and an ELISA. There is generally a good
correlation between the potency as determined with in vitro
methods and the efficacy of the vaccine in the field. However,
this correlation is not always perfect. A product with a
sufficiently high antigen content (as determined by in vitro
methods) is sometimes found to induce poor immunity in
quantitative in vivo assays or in a field trial. For this reason,
vaccine producers are reluctant* to use in vitro models in the
final potency control on the polyvalent product, so that for the
time being their application will be limited to in-process
control (20) while an animal test will still be required for the
final control.

---

* In this connection it is advisable to include a vaccine of
  known low potency in the validation of in vitro tests, this
  being in contrast with the validating procedure now in common
  use. In this way, the ability of the model to differentiate
  between high- and poor-quality products might be established at
  an early stage.

In the recent past this test was based on a qualitative assay
(antibody response above a fixed value) in monkeys. Most
countries have, however, changed over to a quantitative assay
based on determination of the titre of neutralizing antibodies.
Table 3 lists the guidelines and their specifications for this
test.
All, except the American, guidelines agree on the methodology and
assessment criterion, while they differ as regards the animal
species and the number of animal groups to be used. A comparative
study (23) indicated that the rat is one of the most suitable
animal models for estimating the potency of polio vaccines, with
the exception of the DPT-polio vaccine, this being due to the
pertussis component in this vaccine. Monkeys are therefore still
used for the DPT-polio vaccine.

Table 3: SPECIFICATIONS OF THE EXISTING GUIDELINES FOR
DETERMINING THE POTENCY OF INACTIVATED POLIO VACCINE
(polyvalent vaccine)

Specifications	Distress category 1*					
	WHO (9)	Eur.Ph. (21)	Neth. (6)	UK (22)	USA (7)	Japan (8)
Species	rat	guinea pig/ chicken	rat	guinea pig/ chicken	monkey	-
No. of animal groups	3	3	4	3	1	-
No. of animals/group	≥10	10	10	10	≥12	-
Route of administration	i.m.	i.m.	i.m.	i.m.	i.m.	-
Reference vaccine	yes	n.s.	yes	n.s.	ref. serum	-
- no. of animal groups	3		4			
- no. of animals/group	n.s.		n.s.			
Criterion	.... Serology					

* See chapter 5, section 4
i.m. = intramuscular; n.s. = not specified.
Note: Japan has only guidelines for live polio vaccine.

If in the future the potency test of the diphtheria, tetanus and
pertussis vaccines can be assayed by immunization of mice and
subsequent in vitro antibody titration, then the next logical
step would be to develop a test for the various inactivated
vaccine types which can be performed in one and the same animal
species. Combining several potency assays in one animal model is
a particularly attractive proposition in terms of reducing
laboratory animal use.
Yet another approach might be the validation of an in vitro model
based on antigen-induced antibody systhesis by human lymphocytes.
Preliminary studies showed an antigen-specific and dose-dependent
response for the poliovirus types 1, 2 and 3 (24).

7.A.6. Test for abnormal toxicity
See chapter 8, section 2.3.

7.B. Live, oral poliomyelitis vaccine

Since the early sixties, when most countries replaced the Salk by
the Sabin vaccine, the live, attenuated (Sabin) poliomyelitis
vaccine has been used on a wide scale, usually as a trivalent
product containing poliovirus serotypes 1, 2 and 3 (1). It is
administered orally in the form of a sugar lump. The virus is
propagated for vaccine production in cultures of primary monkey
kidney cells or in human diploid cells. When the latter are used,
an appropriate test in animals is required to ensure freedom from
tumourigenic properties. The recommendations for this test are
the same as those made in section 7.A.4. The routine quality
control tests relevant to the 3-R objectives of this project are:
- test for extraneous agents;
- test for neurovirulence;
- test for abnormal toxicity.

7.B.1. Test for extraneous agents

Several tests are available to check the monovalent virus harvest
or the monovalent virus suspension for freedom from adventitious
microorganisms. The guidelines and specifications for these tests
are summarized in tables 4, 5, 6 and 7.
The purpose of the various tests is:
- test in newborn and adult mice: to demonstrate freedom from
  adventitious agents;
- test in rabbits: to demonstrate freedom from extraneous
  microorganisms, particularly herpesvirus 1;
- test in guinea pigs: to demonstrate freedom from extraneous
  microorganisms, particularly Mycobacterium tuberculosis and LCM
  virus.
When tissues from monkeys bred in captivity under well-controlled
conditions are used as a source of cell substrate, the need for
two tests, i.e. in rabbits and in guinea pigs, may be questioned
for the same reason as given in section 7.A.3.1. for the
inactivated polio vaccine. In addition, an expert group of WHO
consultants has recently reviewed the tests under discussion
here. They concluded that the tests in small laboratory animals
could be dispensed with because these tests do not contribute to
assuring the safety of the vaccine. The ability of these tests to
detect extraneous microorganisms is actually far inferior to that
of the cell cultures system (25). However, the testing of the
virus seed in animals should be continued.

Table 4: SPECIFICATIONS OF THE EXISTING GUIDELINES FOR TESTING
THE ORAL POLIO VACCINE FOR EXTRANEOUS VIRUSES IN GUINEA
PIGS

| Specifications | Distress category 1* | | |
	WHO (25)	USA (7)	Japan (8)
Species	guinea pig	guinea pig	guinea pig
No. of animals	5	5	5
Route of administration	i.p.	i.p.	i.p.+i.c.
Observation period (days)	42	42	42
Criterion	.... Clinical symptoms		
	.... microscopic changes		

* see chapter 5, section 4
i.p. = intraperitoneal   i.c. = intracerebral

Table 5: SPECIFICATIONS OF THE EXISTING GUIDELINES FOR TESTING
THE ORAL POLIO VACCINE FOR EXTRANEOUS VIRUSES IN RABBITS

Specifications	Distress category 1*		
	WHO (25)	USA (7)	Japan (8)
Species	rabbit	rabbit	rabbit
No. of animals	10	10	10
Route of administration	s.c.+i.d.	s.c.+i.d.	s.c.+i.d.
Observation period (weeks)	3	3	3
Criterion	.... Clinical symptoms		
	.... microscopic changes		

* see chapter 5, section 4
s.c. = subcutaneous   i.d. = intradermal

Table 6: SPECIFICATIONS OF THE EXISTING GUIDELINES FOR TESTING
THE ORAL POLIO VACCINE FOR EXTRANEOUS VIRUSES IN ADULT
MICE

Specifications	Distress category 1*		
	WHO (25)	USA (7)	Japan (8)
Species	mouse	mouse	mouse
No. of animals	20	20	20
Route of administration	i.c+i.p.	i.c.+i.p.	i.c.+i.p.
Observation period (weeks)	3	3	3
Criterion	.... Clinical symptoms		
	.... microscopic changes		

* see chapter 5, section 4
i.p. = intraperitoneal   i.c. = intracerebral

Table 7: SPECIFICATIONS OF THE EXISTING GUIDELINES FOR TESTING
THE ORAL POLIO VACCINE FOR EXTRANEOUS VIRUSES IN NEWBORN
MICE

Specifications	Distress category 1*		
	WHO (25)	USA (7)	Japan (8)
Species	mouse	mouse	mouse
No. of animals	10	20	10
Route of administration	i.c+i.p.	i.c.+i.p.	i.c.+i.p.
Observation period (weeks)	2	2	2
Criterion	.... Clinical symptoms		
	.... microscopic changes		

* see chapter 5, section 4
i.p. = intraperitoneal   i.c. = intracerebral

7.B.2. <u>Test for neurovirulence</u>
The poliovirus is a neurotropic virus. Although the virus is
attenuated, a small number of polio-associated paralytic cases
occur every year. The estimated incidence is less than one case
per million oral vaccine recipients (26). Six or seven cases per
year were reported in the U.S. in the period 1980-1982 (27). The
polio virus can occasionally revert to neurovirulence. Each
poliovirus type must therefore be checked for neurovirulence
before the vaccine can be considered for use in man. The only
known animal species which can be used to predict neurovirulence
is the monkey (Rhesus or Cynomolgus monkeys).
In the neurovirulence test, samples of the bulk virus suspension
produced are injected into a group of monkeys in the lumbar
region of the spinal cord and in most countries also in the right
and left thalamic regions of the brain. Another group of animals
is similarly inoculated with a reference preparation and serves
as a control group. The specifications of the various guidelines
for the neurovirulence test are listed in table 8.

Table 8: THE GUIDELINES AND THEIR SPECIFICATIONS FOR THE
NEUROVIRULENCE TEST ON ORAL POLIO VACCINE

Specifications	Distress category 5*			
	WHO (25)	USA (7)	UK (28)	Japan (8)
Species	monkey (r or c)	monkey (r)	monkey (c)	monkey (r)
No. of animal groups	1	4	4	7
No. of animals/group	type 1:12 type 2:12 type 3:20	each virus type:45	each virus type:45	each virus type:45
Route of administration	i.s.	i.c.+i.s.	i.c.+i.s.	i.c.+i.s
Observation period (days)	17-22	17-22		18
Reference preparation	yes	yes	yes	yes
- no. of animal groups	1	4	4	7
- no. of animals/group	type 1,2:12 type 3:20	each virus type:45	each virus type:45	each virus type:45
Criterion	. Clinical and histopathological findings.			

* = See chapter 5, section 4
i.c. = intracerebral   i.s. = intraspinal
type = virus type   r   = Rhesus   c = Cynomolgus

It shows that there are marked differences as to the recommended
test procedure, the species of monkey used, the number of animal
groups, and the number of animals used per group. For example,
only the WHO guidelines do not specify intracerebral
administration of the virus suspension. Furthermore, the total
number of animal groups for each experiment (that is, for the
virus type being tested plus the reference preparation) varies
from 2 (WHO) to 14 (Japan), so that the total number of animals
required for each virus type lies between 24 (WHO, virus types 1
and 2) and 90 (Japan). The reason for these differences is that
opinions differ widely on several aspects of the test procedure.
For example, the U.S. attaches greater value to the results from
the intracerebral test than to those from the intraspinal test,

whereas the U.K. takes the opposing view (28). The Japanese
regulations recommend a five-dilution method for determining
neurovirulence (26), whereas the WHO considers a single virus
concentration to be sufficient. In 1982 the WHO stated, on the
basis of the results of a collaborative project consisting of
experiments and retrospective analysis of oral polio vaccine
testing over the preceding 18 years, that neither the
intracerebral nor the intraspinal test makes the best use of
monkeys (25). Their reason, in the case of the intracerebral test
was the monkey's relative insusceptibility to the virus, and in
that of the intraspinal test, the insensitivity of the assessment
criterion used.
The WHO Expert Group concluded that an intraspinal test can
provide the information required for making an accurate
comparison of a virus type with the appropriate reference
preparation, using only a small number of monkeys, the assessment
criterion being the distribution of virus-specific lesions within
the central nervous system (25). It seems therefore justified to
bring the various national specifications for the neurovirulence
test into line with those of the WHO. Since there is no immediate
prospect for an in vitro approach to the neurovirulence test, the
WHO method mentioned above is the best model from the viewpoint
of the 3-R objectives.

7.B.3. Test for abnormal toxicity
See chapter 8, section 2.3.

8. RABIES VACCINE

Most countries use an inactivated rabies vaccine for active
immunization against rabies. In the Netherlands the virus is
grown in microcarrier culture of primary dog kidney cells. The
following aspects of the production and control of the rabies
vaccine are relevant to the 3-R objectives of this project:
- production;
- test for residual live virus;
- test for extraneous agents;
- potency test;
- test for abnormal toxicity.

8.1. Production
The rabies vaccine is one of the earliest vaccine products made.
The in vivo virus culturing technique introduced by Pasteur has
long been used for the production of rabies vaccine, although it
has undergone modifications over the years. The substrates for
virus cultivation that have been described and are still used
today in some countries include the brains of sheep, newborn mice
and newborn rabbits (29).
Although in vitro culture has recently also become possible, some
countries still cultivate the virus in vivo. This alternative
approach not only led to a reduction in animal usage but it also
lowered the risk of neurological complications associated with
the use of in vivo produced vaccines. In vitro produced vaccines
are generally safe and effective.
Only one dog is used in the Netherlands for obtaining the primary
kidney cells needed for growing the vaccine virus (30). The other
cell substrates for production purposes reported in the
literature include various diploid cell lines (31, 32), rabbit
embryo fibroblasts (FEL cells) (33) and chick embryo cells (PCEC
cells) (34).

The problem with diploid cell lines for virus propagation is that large-scale production is not possible. Generally good results have been reported with the other cell substrates. However, changing over to a new cell line for cultivation of the virus normally requires extensive validation and is very expensive, so that it is not realistic within the framework of this project to make recommendations on this here.

8.2. Test for residual live virus

The rabies virus is inactivated with propiolactone. To detect any incompletely inactivated rabies virus, the liquid vaccine is tested both in vitro (tissue culture) and in vivo. Table 9 summarizes the guidelines and their specifications for the in vivo test. There are two reasons which make it desirable to validate the relevance of this in vivo model, namely:
- it may be questioned whether the in vivo test is more sensitive than the tissue culture test, partly in view of the remarks made about this test for the polio vaccine concerning the sample volume (chapter 6, section 2.5.);
- also, the rabies virus used (at least in the Netherlands) for vaccination purposes has only a limited virulence for man. Even if infectious rabies virus is still present in the vaccine, this will not give rise to clinical symptoms in man.

Table 9: GUIDELINES AND THEIR SPECIFICATIONS FOR THE TEST FOR
RESIDUAL LIVE VIRUS ON RABIES VACCINE

	Distress category 1*			
Specifications	WHO (35)	Neth.(6)	UK (22)	Japan (8)
Species	mouse/ rabbit/ guinea pig	mouse	mouse	mouse/ rabbit
No. of animal groups	1	1	1	1
No. of animals/group	20 mice/ 3 rabbits	20	10	10 mice/ 2 rabbits
Route of administration	i.c.	i.c.	i.c.	i.c.
Observation period (days)	n.s.	10	15	21
Criterion	.... Rabies			

* = See chapter 5, section 4
n.s. = not specified   i.c. = intracerebral

8.3. Tests for extraneous microorganisms

In the case of the rabies vaccine, too, this test consists of a combination of serological assays (in the donor animal), tissue culture tests and animal studies.
Animal testing is performed on the crude virus suspension and comprises two specific and two aspecific tests, discussed below.

8.3.1. Test for Mycobacterium tuberculosis

As dog kidney cells derived from animals bred in controlled and closed breeding units are now used for growing the rabies virus, the same reasoning applies to the test for the presence of Mycobacterium tuberculosis in the rabies vaccine as to this test on the measles vaccine (section 6.1.1. of this chapter).

8.3.2. <u>Tests for extraneous viruses</u>

8.3.2.1. <u>In dogs</u>
When dog kidney cells are used for culturing the rabies virus
then the test for detection of species-specific viral
contamination is also performed in dogs. Four dogs are injected
intraperitoneally with the neutralized virus suspension, and
subsequently observed for 30 days. None of the dogs should
exhibit signs of the disease during this period. Antibodies to a
number of specified virus species should also be absent. The test
usually causes little distress to the animals, and the same
animals are normally used for this test for many years. The
relevance of both the test in dogs and that in mice (section
8.3.2.2.) can be questioned in the case of the inactivated
vaccine (see for a discussion section 7.A.3.2).

8.3.2.2. <u>In mice</u>
See section 7.A.3.2. for the design and execution of this test
and relevant remarks.

8.4. <u>Potency test</u>
The NIH (National Institutes of Health (Bethesda, USA)) mouse
protection test is in general use for estimating the potency of
the rabies vaccine. In this quantitative assay, the potency of
the vaccine under examination is compared with that of a
reference vaccine, the endpoint being death following challenge
with the virulent virus. Table 10 lists the existing guidelines
and specifications for this test.

Table 10: GUIDELINES AND THEIR SPECIFICATIONS FOR THE POTENCY
TEST ON RABIES VACCINE

| Specifications | Distress category 4* | | | | |
	WHO** (35)	Eur.Ph. (21)	Neth. (6)	UK (22)	Japan (8)
Species	mouse	mouse	mouse	mouse	mouse
No. of animal groups	n.s.	3	3	3	5
No. of animals/group		16	20	16	≥10
Route of administration	n.s.	i.p.	i.p.	i.p.	i.p.
Duration:					
- immunization (days)		14	14	14	14
- assessment after					
challenge (days)		14	14	14	14
Control group	n.s.	yes	yes	yes	yes
- no. of animal groups		4	4	4	≥3
- no. of animals/group		10	8	10	10
Reference vaccine	yes	yes	yes	yes	n.s.
Mode of challenge	n.s.	i.c.	i.c.	i.c.	i.c.
- no. of animal groups		3	3	3	
Criterion	.... Death				

* See chapter 5, section 4
** Requirements for rabies vaccine produced in continuous cell
lines.
n.s. = not specified;
i.p. = intraperitoneal;   i.c. = intracerebral.

All, except the Japanese, guidelines broadly agree on the design and execution of this test. Nevertheless, the test is generally considered to be far from ideal, for the following reasons:
- it does not distinguish satisfactorily between different vaccine products as regards their potency (35);
- it gives widely differing results for the same vaccine in different laboratories;
- it is expensive, time-consuming and requires many animals which, moreover suffer considerable pain and distress.

Alternative methods have been reported, such as antibody determination in mice (36) as well as in vitro methods such as single radial immunodiffusion (SRD) and ELISA. The in vitro methods can be standardized well, make an accurate determination possible and give a good correlation with the NIH potency test. However, the application of in vitro methods is as yet limited to in-process control. If in the potency testing of the first few vaccine batches of a new vaccine strain a good correlation has been found to exist between the in vivo and the in vitro methods, an in vitro potency assay could then be used for testing the subsequent batches derived from the same strain. Another in vitro assay, the antibody binding test (ABT) (40, 41), holds better prospects. In this quantitative assay, a vaccine dilution is mixed with an equal volume of neutralizing antiserum, to which an indicator (rabies) virus is added. Next, a chick embryo fibroblast culture is inoculated with this vaccine-serum-virus mixture. After an incubation period of 3 days and the subsequent addition of fluorescent antiglobulin, fluorescent foci appear in the culture depending on the amount of unneutralized virus present. The potency of the product can be expressed in international units if a standard preparation is included in the assay.

The reliability of this test has been validated in comparison with the NIH mouse protection test. It was found that the ABT gives better results than the NIH test as regards variability, reliability and reproducibility.

The ABT is now used for in-process control in some countries; an in vivo method is still stipulated for the final quality control. On the basis of the above, a greater use of the ABT in potency testing could well be considered. The rabies vaccine is a monovalent product. Few ingredients are added to the vaccine which can appreciably affect its potency. This offers the possibility of determining the potency of the first batches (e.g. the first five) produced with a new master seed virus by the mouse protection test and to use the ABT for the following batches, provided that a positive correlation has been demonstrated between the two methods.

Yet another approach to measuring the potency of the rabies vaccine is in vitro lymphocyte stimulation. In accordance with the remarks made in chapter 8, section 7.5., this model offers a promising alternative (42) and further study is worthwhile.

8.5. Test for abnormal toxicity

See chapter 8, section 2.3. for the characteristics of this test and recommendations.

9. RUBELLA VACCINE

A live attenuated virus is used for active immunization, propagated in primary rabbit or dog kidney cells, or in human diploid cells. The following aspects of rubella vaccine

production and control are relevant to the 3-R objectives of this project:
- tests for extraneous agents;
- test for abnormal toxicity.

9.1. Production
The conventional way of culturing the rubella virus is in primary rabbit kidney cells. In 1987, however, the Netherlands began to use diploid cells for this purpose (43). Apart from the fact that as a result rabbits are no longer needed for production of the vaccine virus, this change also had two consequences for the in vivo tests, namely:
- when diploid cells are used, the current WHO guidelines stipulate batch testing of the production cells for tumourigenic properties;
- also, testing for extraneous viruses can - as far as the animal tests are concerned - be restricted to the "master cell bank", the stock of cells from which the production cells are derived.

9.2. Tests for extraneous agents
See section 6.1. on the measles vaccine for a description of the test for freedom from Mycobacterium tuberculosis and extraneous viruses, and relevant remarks. In addition, there is in the Netherlands a test for the detection of species-specific viral contamination. It is performed in 5 rabbits and is based on a serological assessment following intradermal and subcutaneous administration of the virus suspension. With the introduction of the new substrate cells this test will be discontinued.

9.3. Abnormal-toxicity test
See chapter 8, section 2.3. for particulars of this test, and recommendations.

10. SUMMARY

The following approaches towards reduction or refinement of laboratory animal use in the production and quality control of human viral vaccines can be, or have recently been, implemented.

In the short term (within 5 years)
- GENERAL:
  - reduction in the number of animals for the abnormal-toxicity test;
  - discontinuation of the test for Mycobacterium tuberculosis when animals are used from closed breeding units and GMP rules are implemented.

- INACTIVATED POLIO VACCINE
  - Production:
    - increase the cell harvest per animal by improvement of the perfusion technique;
    - use of Vero cells instead of tertiary monkey kidney cells.
  - Inactivation:
    - replacement of the test for residual live virus in monkeys by a test in tissue culture (this is already a fact in most countries);
    - substitution of Vero cells for tertiary monkey kidney cells.

- Extraneous viruses: - discontinuation of the test in
                        laboratory animals.

- LIVE ATTENUATED POLIO VACCINE
  - Extraneous viruses: - discontinuation of the tests in
                          laboratory animals.
  - Neurovirulence: - harmonization of the various national
                          guidelines for this test with those of
                          the WHO.

- RABIES VACCINE
  - Inactivation: - discontinuation of the test in
                          laboratory animals.

  - Extraneous viruses: - discontinuation of the tests in
                          laboratory animals.
  - Potency test: - replacement of the lethal intracerebral
                          challenge by an immunological assay
                          (the ABT or ELISA).

- RUBELLA VACCCINE
  - Production: - replacement of propagation in rabbit
                          kidney cells by cultivation in diploid
                          cells.

In the medium term (5-10 years)
- LIVE VACCINES IN GENERAL
  - possible replacement of the animal models for the test for
    extraneous viruses by tissue culture systems.

- POLIO VACCINE
  - Production: - cultivation of the virus in continuous
                          cell lines.

- GENERAL
  - introduction of novel techniques, making it highly likely
    that more uniform vaccines can be produced, which will in
    turn reduce the extent of quality control (see chapter 13);
  - replacement of the immunization part of the in vivo model for
    potency testing by an in vitro method based on lymphocyte
    stimulation (see recommendations made for the diphtheria
    vaccine in chapter 8, section 4.3.3.);
  - validation of in vitro alternatives for the tumourigenicity
    test.

11. REFERENCES

1. Marten, M.: The price of polio vaccine. Lab. Anim. (1981), 10, (1), 20-25
2. Levenbuk, J.S. et al.: On the morphological evaluation of the neurovirulence safety of attenuated mumps virus strains in monkeys. Journ. Biol. Standard. (1977), 7, 9-19
3. W.H.O.: Technical Report Series 725, (1985)
4. Wood, J.M. et al.: International collaborative study of single-radial-diffusion and immunoelectrophoresis techniques for the assay of haemagglutinin antigen of influenza virus. Journ. Biol. Standard. (1981), 9, 317-330
5. W.H.O.: Technical Report Series 329, (1966)
6. Werkvoorschriften Virusvaccins RIVM. (Specifications for the viral vaccines.) RIVM, the Netherlands, 1983
7. Code of Federal Regulations, FDA, No. 21, 600-799, (1982)
8. Minimum requirement of biological products. Ministry of Health and Welfare, Japanese Government, (1982)
9. W.H.O.: Technical Report Series 673, (1982)
10. Hennessen, W.: Replacement of animals in manufacture and control of vaccines. Develop. Biol. Standard. (1980), 45,163-173
11. Kruijt, B.C.: Personal communication
12. Montagnon, B.J. et al.: The large scale cultivation of VERO-cells in micro-carrier culture for virus vaccine production; preliminary results for killed poliovirus vaccine. Develop. Biol. Standard. (1981), 47, 55-64
13. Beale, A.J.: Cell substrate for killed polio vaccine production. Develop. Biol. Standard. (1981), 47, 19-23
14. Levenbook, J.S. et al.: Tumorigenicity of VERO-cells. Journ. Biol. Standard. (1984), 12, 391-398
15. Steenis, G. van and Wezel, A.L. van: Killed polio vaccine: an evaluation of safety testing. Develop. Biol. Standard. (1981), 47, 143-151
16. Steenis, G. van and Wezel, A.L. van: Use of the ATG-treated newborn rat for in vivo tumorigenicity testing of cell substrates. Develop. Biol. Standard. (1982), 50, 37-46
17. Bather, R. et al.: Heterotransplantation studies with tissueculture cell lines in various animal and in vitro host systems. Journ. Biol. Standard. (1985), 13, 13-23
18. Noguchi, P.D. et al.: Chick embryonic skin as a rapid organ culture assay for cellular neoplasia. Science (1978), 199, 980-983
19. Levenbook, J.S. et al.: Tumorigenicity testing of primate cell lines in nude mice, muscle organ culture and for colony formation in soft agarose. Journ. Biol. Standard. (1985), 13, 135-141
20. Seefried, A. von et al.: Comparisons of poliovirus antigen measurements in vitro and in small animals. Develop. Biol. Standard. (1981), 47, 91-100
21. European Pharmacopoeia, Mon. 216, (1983)
22. British Pharmacopoeia, Vol. II, (1980)
23. Steenis, G. van et al.: Potency testing of killed polio vaccine in rats. Develop. Biol. Standard. (1981), 47, 119-128
24. UytdeHaag, F.G.C.M. et al.: Human peripheral blood lymphocytes from recently vaccinated individuals produce both type-specific and intertypic cross reacting neutralizing antibody on in vitro stimulation with one type of poliovirus. The Journal of Immunology (1985), 135, 5, 3094-3101
25. W.H.O.: Technical Report Series 687, (1983)

26. Chino, F. et al.: Evaluation of the neurovirulence test of oral poliovaccines in Japan during the period 1963-1982. Japan. J. Med. Sci. Biol. (1984), 37, 233-240
27. Schonberger, L.B. et al.: Control of Paralytic Poliomyelitis in the United States. Reviews Inf. Dis. (1984), 6, Suppl. 2, S424-S426
28. Elisberg, B.L.: Standardization of Safety and Potency tests of Vaccines Against Poliomyelitis. Reviews Inf. Dis. (1984), 6, Suppl. 2, S519-S522
29. Steenis, G. van et al.: Nederlands celkweekrabies vaccin voor toepassing bij de mens. (Dutch cell-cultured rabies vaccine for use in man) Ned. Tijdschr. Geneeskd. (1984), 128, 28, 1810-1814
30. Kruijt, B.C.: Personal communication
31. Berlin, B.S. et al.: Rhesus diploid rabies vaccine (adsorbed). A new rabies vaccine. JAMA, 247, 12, (1982), 1726-1728
32. Burgoyne, G.H. et al.: Rhesus diploid rabies vaccine (adsorbed). A new rabies vaccine using FRhL-2 cells. Journ. Infect. Dis. (1985), 152, 1, 204-210
33. Sureau, P. et al.: A rabies vaccine produced in a non-tumorigenic rabbit cell line. Develop. Biol. Standard. (1985), 60, 133-139
34. Barth, R. et al.: A new inactivated tissue culture rabies vaccine for use in man. Evaluation of PCEC-vaccine by laboratory tests. Journ. Biol. Standard. (1984), 12, 29-46
35. W.H.O.: Technical Report Series 760, (1987)
36. Rosanoff, E.J.: The potency of rabies vaccines as determined by the induction of antibody in mice. Journ. Biol. Standard. (1979), 7, 1-7
37. Ferguson, M. et al.: Single radial diffusion assays for the standardization of the antigenic content of rabies vaccines. Develop. Biol. Standard. (1986), 64, 81-86
38. Fitzgerald, E.A. and Needy, C.F.: Use of the single radial immunodiffusion test as a replacement for the NIH mouse potency test for rabies vaccine. Develop. Biol. Standard. (1986), 64, 73-79
39. Adamovicz, P. et al.: The use of various immunochemical, biochemical and biological methods for the analysis of rabies virus production in tissue cultures. Develop. Biol. Standard. (1984), 55, 191-197
40. Barth, R. et al.: The antibody-binding test, a useful method for quantitative determination of inactivated rabies virus antigen. Journ. Biol. Standard. (1981), 9, 81-89
41. Barth, R. et al.: Validation of an in vitro assay for the determination of rabies antigen. Develop. Biol. Standard. (1986), 64, 87-92
42. UytdeHaag, F.G.C.M. et al.: Induction of antigen-specific antibody response in human peripheral blood lymphocytes in vitro by a dog kidney cell vaccine against rabies virus (DKCV). The Journal of Immunology (1983), 131, 3, 1234-1239
43. Steenis, G. van: Personal communication

CHAPTER 10: OPPORTUNITIES FOR REPLACEMENT, REDUCTION OR REFINEMENT: POULTRY VACCINES

1. INTRODUCTION

Many millions of poultry are reared for egg and meat production in the Netherlands every year. These birds usually spend their entire life in an indoor environment where the risk of infection ("infection pressure") is always high. Keeping large numbers of birds under such conditions would not be possible without adequate prophylaxis against several infectious diseases. For this reason active immunization plays a major part in the veterinary care of the poultry stock.
Several poultry vaccines are made in the Netherlands on an industrial scale. Most of these products are of viral origin, and the design and execution of the animal tests on them are broadly similar. This discussion can therefore be confined to the individual animal tests. They can be divided into two groups, namely, in vivo tests on live, attenuated poultry vaccines and in vivo tests on inactivated poultry vaccines.

2. LIVE, ATTENUATED POULTRY VACCINES

Live, attenuated vaccines are attractive for the vaccination of large numbers, because these vaccines can be given in the drinking water, whereas inactivated vaccines must be administered to each individual bird. Many poultry vaccines are therefore based on a live attenuated virus strain. The vaccines against the following avian diseases are concerned here:
- avian encephalomyelitis (AE);
- avian infectious bursal disease (IBD, or Gumboro disease);
- avian infectious bronchitis (IB);
- avian infectious laryngotracheitis (ILT);
- Marek's disease;
- Newcastle disease (NCD);
- fowl pox.
The vaccines are normally produced by growing the seed virus in embryonated hen's eggs or in chick embryo cell cultures. The in vivo tests are all carried out in the species for which the vaccine is intended (the target species).
The principal animal tests included in the quality control of vaccines batches are the test for extraneous microorganisms and the safety test. An in vivo potency test is required for only one representative batch of a seed lot, and usually involves a lethal challenge. An in vitro assay, based on virus titration, is sufficient for the other vaccine batches prepared from the same seed lot. (Note: in a few cases this titration is carried out in chick embryos or chicks).
The following table lists the tests for the routine quality control of each vaccine, together with the possibilities of using alternative methods. Not included are the animal tests on the seed lot, which are performed very infrequently. The individual quality control tests are discussed separately, and a summary concludes the chapter.

115

virus titration	test for freedom from virulent poxvirus	identity test	safety test	test for contamination with AE virus	test for contamination with extraneous agents	
±	0	-	+	0	+	Avian encephalomyelitis vaccine
0	0	0	+	±	+	Avian infectious bronchitis vaccine
+	-	0	+	±	+	Fowlpox vaccine
0	0	0	+	±	+	Avian infectious bursal disease vaccine
0	0	0	+	±	+	Avian infectious laryngotracheitis vaccine
0	0	0	+	±	+	Vaccine against Marek's disease
0	0	-	+	±	+	Vaccine against Newcastle disease

See chapter 8, table 1 for a key to the symbols.

2.1. Tests for contamination with extraneous agents

The materials (embryonated eggs, cells) used as substrates for
the production of poultry vaccines are derived from the same
animal species as that for which the vaccine is intended. This
homologous vaccine production procedure makes high demands on the
test for possible microbial contamination of the product. Most
guidelines include specifications for this examination, usually
consisting of six complementary tests:
- test for extraneous agents in chicks;
- test for contamination with AE virus in chick embryos or in
  day-old chicks;
- test on culture media for contaminating bacteria, fungi and
  mycoplasmas;
- general test for extraneous viruses in cell cultures;
- specific test for extraneous viruses in cell cultures;
- test for extraneous viruses in embryonated hen's eggs.

The two animal tests feature prominently in the routine quality
control for foreign viruses because the latest guidelines of the
European Pharmacopoeia, for the IB and NCD vaccines (1985),
attach special value to the in vivo tests for this examination.

2.1.1. Test for extraneous agents in chicks

Unless mentioned otherwise, the vaccine is administered to a
group of two-week-old chicks by different routes. No clinical
symptoms should develop during the observation period of 5 to 6
weeks nor should the birds' serum contain antibodies to a number
of specified pathogenic viruses (except to the vaccine virus), to
three mycoplasma species, and to Salmonella pullorum. Table 1
summarizes the guidelines and their specifications for this test.
There is agreement on the number of animal groups, the assessment
criteria and the length of the observation period. Differences
exist as to the number of chickens per group, the routes of
administration and the frequency of taking blood samples.

Table 1: GUIDELINES AND THEIR SPECIFICATIONS FOR THE TEST FOR
         EXTRANEOUS AGENTS USING CHICKS

Specifications	A	B	C	Distress category 2* Eur.Ph. (1)	UK (2)	UK-WhB (3)
Species	c	c	c	c	c	c
No. of animal groups	1	1	1	1	1	1
No. of birds/group	13	12	30	≥10	20	≥10
Route of administration	i.m.+ o.c.	i.a.+ i.m + i.n.+ i.t.	i.m.+ o.c.+ i.a.+ i.n.	i.m.+ o.c.	i.m.+ o.c.+ i.a.+ i.n.	i.m.+ o.c.+ i.a.+ i.n.
Frequency of administration	2x	2x	2x	2x	2x	2x
Observation period (weeks)	5	6	6	5	6	6
Days on which blood is taken	0-35	0-21- 42	0-21- 42	0-35	0-21- 42	0-21- 42
Criterion	.... Serology and clinical symptoms					

*   See chapter 5, section 4
WhB = White Book
c   = chicken;   i.a. = intra-articular;
i.m. = intramuscular;   i.n. = intranasal;
o.c. = ocular   i.t. = intrathoracic

Note: - A, B and C represent the specifications of three Dutch
        vaccine manufacturers.
      - To date, the European Pharmacopoeia specifications apply
        officially only to the IB and NCD vaccines. It is
        expected that they will also become mandatory for the
        other live poultry vaccines.

The reason that manufacturer C uses more birds per group than the
guidelines in this table specify is that the manufacturers adjust
their specifications to the guidelines and requirements of the
countries to which they export. When these guidelines do not
agree then more animals may be used than is necessary. This
particular manufacturer exports to a country where 20 animals are
required for the test for extraneous agents, and also to a
country which stipulates that a proportion of the animals be
killed and autopsied at various times during the test. This
example highlights the need for international harmonization of
the guidelines in the interest of achieving an effective
reduction in the usage of animals. Slow progress is now being
made in this field in Europe, to which the publication of the
European Pharmacopoeia monographs has made a positive
contribution.
Because of the binding nature of the European Pharmacopoeia
within Europe, its guidelines are the most relevant for European
countries when testing the different poultry vaccines available.
As regards the objectives of this project - replacement,
reduction, refinement - both a positive and a negative judgement
can be made about the European Pharmacopoeia guideline for the
test for extraneous agents. The positive point is that, compared
with the other existing guidelines, the requirements formulated

in this guideline represent an improvement in conditions for the experimental bird, particularly as regards the pain and distress caused. Intrathoracic, intra-articular and intranasal administration is no longer stipulated and the number of blood samples to be taken is limited to two. This brings the European Pharmacopoeia guideline into more conformity with the prevailing attitudes than, for example, the British (1977) guidelines (5, 6). A further refinement of the test procedure could be achieved by not taking blood at the beginning of the experiment. As a rule, the birds used are derived from controlled and specific pathogen-free (SPF) flocks so that their health status is known at the start of the test. This obviates the need for taking a blood sample for the quality control of the animals.

The negative point is as follows: there are three ways of testing for extraneous microorganisms, namely, in tissue culture, in embryonated hen's eggs, and in vivo. The European Pharmacopoeia stipulates a combination of all three for testing the first batch of a seed lot. The tests in tissue culture and in embryonated eggs though not the in vivo test can then be omitted for routine batch control. The most important point here is that the vaccine virus need not be inactivated for the in vivo study, unlike in the tests in cell cultures and embryonated eggs.

Pragmatically, this fact makes the animal test system the most suitable for testing these vaccines for foreign microorganisms. However, since monospecific antisera are becoming increasingly available and thereby the possibility of vaccine virus neutralization, it seems useful to validate the sensitivity of the animal model in relation to the cell culture and embryonated egg systems, because such data do not yet exist. On the basis of the results, a motivational approach can then be followed in selecting the most relevant model for each vaccine type.

2.1.2. Test for contamination with avian encephalomyelitis virus in chick embryos or day-old chicks

Avian encephalomyelitis (AE) is a disease affecting chiefly young chicks, causing neurological symptoms. The disease is usually subclinical in older birds. However, the virus is transmitted through the egg ("vertical transmission"), and is thus a potential risk of contamination when the eggs are used for the production of various poultry vaccines. Each batch of live vaccine must therefore be tested for freedom from contamination by AE virus, for which there are two officially recognized methods:

- a group of day-old chicks is inoculated intracerebrally with the vaccine and then checked for signs of AE during the following three weeks;
- the vaccine is injected into the yolk sac of a number of 5 to 7-day-old SPF embryos; the embryos are hatched and the chicks observed for 15 days. The chicks should remain free from signs of AE during the observation period.

Table 2 lists the specifications of the existing guidelines for this test. The guidelines are in broad agreement on the testing procedure, but there are nevertheless doubts about the method's reliability (9, 10), partly because of the possibility of aspecific reactions and partly because only one dose is used. The results of a comparative study (11) into several alternative approaches have recently been published, viz., an in vitro test in chicken embryo brain cell cultures, an in vivo test in day-old chicks (serological assessment), and an in vivo test in 14-day-old chicks (serological assessment). These results indicated

that the in vitro assay is less sensitive than the in vivo assays.
Of the latter, the serological test, either agar gel precipitation or an ELISA, in 14-day-old chicks proved to be superior to the officially prescribed tests. This offers the opportunity to incorporate the test for contamination by AE virus into the test for extraneous microorganisms, for the latter is also performed in 14-day-old chicks and is based on a serological assessment. However, more study is needed because several aspects of the serological estimation of the AE virus are not yet clear, such as the sensitivity of the field strains and the immunological technique to be used. The results of this study can contribute to an evaluation by the compilers of the European Pharmacopoeia on the basis of which the guidelines can be adapted.

Table 2: SPECIFICATIONS OF THE EXISTING GUIDELINES FOR TESTING POULTRY VACCINES FOR CONTAMINATION WITH AE VIRUS

Specifications	D	E	F	Eur.Ph. (7)	UK (8)	UK-WhB (3)
			Distress category 2*			
Species	d-o chick	d-o chick	d-o chick	d-o chick	d-o chick	d-o chick
No. of animal groups	1	1	1	1	1	1
No. of birds/group	10	10	≥15	10	10	10
Route of administration	i.c.	i.c.	i.c.	i.c.	i.c.	i.c.
Observation period (weeks)	3	3	2	3	3	3
Criterion	.... Clinical symptoms					

* See chapter 5, section 4
WhB = White Book;   d-o = day-old
i.c. = intracerebral

Note: - D, E and F refer to three Dutch vaccine manufacturers.
      - The specifications may differ slightly as regards the number of chicks required for each vaccine product.

2.2. Safety evaluation
For those poultry vaccines which are tested for safety (e.g. specific toxicity) in the target animal, most pharmacopoeias state that the abnormal-toxicity test may be combined with the safety test.
In this combined test, a group of chickens receives an excess of the vaccine (usually 2 to 10 times the field dose). The age of the birds and the route of administration depend on the manufacturer's specification. The birds are monitored for clinical symptoms during the observation period. Table 3 summarizes the specifications of the various guidelines for this test, in this particular case the safety test on the IB vaccine. The number of birds and the length of the observation period are virtually the same for the other vaccines. There are differences as regards the number of chickens to be used. It is, however, difficult to indicate what the exact number should be.

Table 3: SPECIFICATIONS FOR THE SAFETY TEST ON POULTRY VACCINES

Specifications	G	H	I	Distress category 2* Eur.Ph. (11)	UK (12)	UK-WhB (3)
Species	c	c	c	c	c	c
No. of animal groups	1	1	1	1	1	1
No. of birds/group	25	12	10	≥ 10	10	25
Route of administration	i.n.	i.n.	i.n.	i.n.	i.n.	i.n.
- dose	10-fold	10-fold	10-fold	10-fold	10-fold	10-fold
Observation period (weeks)	3	3	3	3	2	3
Criterion	.... Clinical symptoms					

----

* See chapter 5, section 4
WhB = White Book;   i.n. = intranasal;   c = chick

Note: G, H and I are the specifications of three Dutch
      manufacturers.

Two to three animals are normally used with the veterinary
vaccines for mammals. This suggests that it would be realistic to
reduce the number of chickens used for the safety test on the
poultry vaccine batches.
Another issue concerns the relevance of the safety test. In
general, the reasons for performing this test on vaccines are the
detection of:
- residual virulence of the vaccine virus;
- contamination with endotoxins;
- consequences of overdosage;
- chemical contamination or other accidents during production and
  packaging.
The following remarks are relevant here: any residual virulence
of the vaccine virus is already detected in the test on the
master seed virus. The presence of small amounts of endotoxins in
the vaccine suspension does not actually affect the quality of
the product, because it is administered in the drinking water
which itself is not endotoxin-free. Furthermore, the LAL test can
be used for testing for endotoxins. Regarding the consequences of
overdosage, testing the first few batches of a seed lot should be
sufficient since subsequent batches will not differ much in this
respect. This leaves the possibility of accidents occurring
during production and packaging. This likelihood is the same as
with the human vaccines, and it was recommended here to minimize
the frequency of testing for abnormal toxicity. The same proposal
could therefore be made for the safety test on poultry vaccines.
It is also possible to combine the safety test with the test for
extraneous agents (see section 2.5.) or to combine the safety
test of several vaccine batches in one experiment.

2.3. Titration of the attenuated avian encephalomyelitis vaccine
     virus
The AE virus is titrated in embryonated eggs. The vaccine is
injected into the yolk sac of a number of eggs; some of the eggs
may be kept as controls. The chick embryos and the hatched chicks
are then monitored for clinical AE symptoms during the

observation period. The virus content is calculated from the number of positive chicks. The experimental procedure entails considerable distress for a proportion of the birds. Furthermore, the assay results are variable. A recently reported alternative approach (13, 14) is based on in vitro titration of the virus in cell cultures of chick embryo brain, using indirect fluorescence to reveal the virus. Validation of this method, as well as of the test for contamination with AE virus, is to be recommended.

2.4. Titration of the attenuated fowlpox vaccine virus

In the in vivo determination of the virus titre, groups of about five chickens receive one or more dilutions of the vaccine by the follicle and the wing-web methods. The virus titre is calculated on the basis of clinical symptoms and local post-vaccination reactions.

There are two alternative approaches to this in vivo method:
- titration of the virus in endothelial cell cultures;
- titration in embryonated eggs, the criterion being the development of fowlpox on the egg membrane after inoculation.

One of the Dutch manufacturers has gained experience with the embryonated egg system and has reported favourable results.

2.5. General

Apart from the introduction of new techniques, there is another way of reducing the use of experimental animals, viz. by combining in vivo tests. The combination of the test for contamination by AE virus has already been mentioned. Another possibility is combining the test for extraneous agents with the safety test, on condition that the vaccine virus need not first be inactivated. The practicality of this combination also depends on the route of administration, the dose, and housing of the birds. For example, the use of isolators for the test for extraneous microorganisms can interfere with the detection of clinical symptoms in the safety test. However, this need not stand in the way of combining the safety test and the test for extraneous agents.

3. INACTIVATED POULTRY VACCINES

Among the poultry vaccines, the inactivated vaccines constitute a minority, and only the following four are produced on a routine basis in the Netherlands:
- avian infectious bursal disease (IBD or Gumboro disease) vaccine;
- avian infectious bronchitis (IB) vaccine;
- egg drop syndrome (EDS) vaccine;
- Newcastle disease (NCD) vaccine.

Unlike the live poultry vaccines and both the live and inactivated human virus vaccines, no in vivo tests for freedom from extraneous microorganisms are required in the quality control of the inactivated poultry vaccines. On the other hand, the potency test and the safety test are an integral part of their quality control. The potency test generally consists of a qualitative or quantitative serological response assay and, in the case of the NCD vaccine, of a lethal challenge. The safety test is similar to that for the live poultry vaccines.

As regards the 3-R objectives of this project, it is difficult to put forward any specific proposals for these tests on the individual vaccines, because official guidelines for these tests, for example, in the European Pharmacopoeia, do not exist yet.

However, several general recommendations can be made, chiefly concerning the potential for combining the tests.

3.1. Testing the potency of two or more vaccines in a single experiment

Opportunities for this exist with those products where the serological response of the chickens is used as the assessment criterion of the potency test, in this case the IB, IBD and EDS vaccines. It can lead to a considerable reduction in the number of birds required for testing these vaccines. However, one consequence is that the animals used for the combined test suffer more distress than before, because of the greater frequency of vaccine administration and blood withdrawal. The feasibility of this approach depends on the production planning of the individual vaccines and on the stipulations of the regulatory authorities for this test. Furthermore, a validation procedure will have to be carried out to find out whether there is any interaction between the vaccines involved in the combined test.

3.2. Combining the potency test and the safety test

To date, this possibility has been hampered by the fact that the specifications differ as to the vaccine doses to be used in these tests, this being one dose or less for the potency test and a double dose for the safety test. Opinions differ on the latter. It is desirable to investigate what effect a reduction of the dose has on the value of the safety test.

3.3. Sequential testing

Another way to reduce the number of chickens required is to perform several tests in sequence, using the same group of animals. An example is the potency test based on a serological assessment. It is theoretically possible to use the same birds for different vaccines. However, one difficulty is that the guidelines generally specify the age of the chickens to be used so that, if sequential testing is employed, the birds will often be too old for one or more tests. It can be questioned whether the age specifications are equally relevant in all cases. They should be examined more closely before sequential testing can be considered for application. However, it should also be realized that sequential testing causes greater distress to the animals concerned. It will therefore be necessary to weigh the pros and cons of this approach.

4. SUMMARY

The following recommendations can be made for reducing or refining the use of experimental animals for the quality control of poultry vaccines.

A) Live attenuated vaccines
- TEST FOR EXTRANEOUS AGENTS IN CHICKS:
  - bringing the guidelines into line with those of the European Pharmacopoeia for the IB and NCD vaccines;
  - discontinuation of blood sampling at the beginning of the test;
  - evaluation of the in vivo test with respect to the tests in tissue culture and embryonated hen's eggs.

- TEST FOR CONTAMINATION WITH AE VIRUS IN DAY-OLD CHICKS OR CHICK EMBRYOS:
  - introduction of an alternative approach based on serological assessment in two-week-old chicks and combining this test with the test for extraneous agents.

- SAFETY TEST:
  - reduction of the number of chickens;
  - re-appraisal of the need for this test.

- TITRATION OF LIVE AE VACCINE VIRUS:
  - validation of an alternative approach in tissue culture.

- TITRATION OF LIVE FOWLPOX VACCINE VIRUS:
  - replacement of the in vivo test by titration in tissue culture or in embryonated hen's eggs.

- GENERAL:
  - combining the safety test with the test for extraneous agents or combining several safety tests in one experiment.

B) Inactivated poultry vaccines
- SAFETY TEST:
  - as stated for live poultry vaccines;
  - re-evaluation of the specifications for the dose to be used.

- GENERAL:
  - combining the potency tests of different vaccines in a single procedure;
  - combining the potency test with the safety test if the results of the re-evaluation of the dose to be used for the latter are positive;
  - introduction of the sequential test if an evaluation of the age requirements and a consideration of the ethical aspects permit.

5. REFERENCES

1. European Pharmacopoeia, V.2.1.3.5, (1983)
2. British Pharmacopoeia (Vet), 1977
3. Ministry of Agriculture, Fisheries and Food, (1977). Specifications for the production and control of avian live virus vaccines. 2nd edition, Ministry of Agriculture, Fisheries and Food, Pinner, U.K.
4. Code of Federal Regulations, F.D.A., (1984), 9, USA
5. Thornton, D.H. et al.: Development of in vitro tests for detection of extraneous agents. Develop. Biol. Standard. (1986), 64, 195-198
6. Wood, S.B. and Wood, G.W.: A comparison of the methods of theEuropean Pharmacopoeia for the detection of Mycoplasma gallisepticum and Mycoplasma synoviae. Journ. Biol. Standard. (1984), 12, 305-309
7. European Pharmacopoeia V2.1.3.2., (1983)
8. British Pharmacopoeia (Vet), (1985)
9. Nicholas, R.A.J. et al.: Studies on the detection of avian encephalomyelitis virus. Research in Veterinary Science, (1986), 40, 118-122
10. Klok, J.: Personal communication
11. European Pharmacopoeia, Mon. 442 (1985)
12. British Pharmacopoeia (Vet) 8, (1977)
13. Berger, R.G.: An in vitro assay for quantifying the virus of avian encephalomyelitis. Avian diseases (1982), 26, 534-541
14. Nicholas, R.A.J. et al.: A comparison of titration methods for live avian encephalomyelitis virus vaccines. Develop. Biol. Standard. (1986), 64, 207-212

CHAPTER 11: OPPORTUNITIES FOR REPLACEMENT, REDUCTION OR
REFINEMENT: VETERINARY VACCINES FOR MAMMALS

1. INTRODUCTION

The veterinary vaccines intended for use in mammals form a rather
heterogeneous group as regards both the range of products
available and the diversity in animal species required for their
quality control, although the latter consists of only a few types
of tests. Thus, the safety test is an integral part of the
quality control of all vaccines; an in vivo potency test is
performed on each batch of the inactivated products but the in
vivo potency testing of nearly all live vaccines is - as with
live poultry vaccines - restricted to one representative batch of
a seed lot. A specific test is stipulated only for the live
attenuated dog vaccines, where each vaccine batch must be checked
for contamination with rabies virus. There are as yet no
international guidelines for a number of products, although
European Pharmacopoeia monographs are in preparation.
The mammalian vaccines produced on a routine basis in the
Netherlands are listed in table 1, together with the relevant
quality control tests. The table also shows where replacement,
reduction or refinement of animal use is already possible or
still under investigation. A few products which are made on only
a small scale have not been included in this list.
This chapter first deals with the general safety test, followed
by a discussion of the other in vivo tests on vaccines for the
individual species. The discussion will be confined to the
existing possibilities of replacement, reduction or refinement of
animal use.

2. SAFETY EVALUATION (general)

For most vaccine products, the safety test is performed on the
species for which the vaccine is intended, i.e., the target
species. Two or three animals are normally used for this test. No
recommendations can be made on a further reduction in this
number. However, it may be considered possible to combine the
safety test with the potency test where both tests are performed
on the target animal and the potency assay is based on serology
rather than on the development of clinical signs and symptoms.
However, the guidelines have so far not permitted such a
combination of tests. This is because of the difference in the
dose specified for the two tests, this being one dose for the
potency test and 2 to 10 doses for the safety test. One reason
for such a high dose was the wish to be able to determine the
consequences of overdosage. When discussing the safety test for
the poultry vaccines (chapter 10, section 2.2.) it was explained
that a test on the seed lot provides enough information on this
point. This means that the administration of an overdose is not
really necessary for routine quality control, so that the amount
of vaccine used can be limited to one dose only. This will make
it possible to combine the safety and potency tests on the
inactivated vaccines. For the inactivated vaccines there is, in
addition to the safety test, also an examination for the absence
of residual virulence of the vaccine strain.

126

Table 1: OPPORTUNITIES FOR REPLACEMENT, REDUCTION AND/OR
REFINEMENT IN THE USE OF EXPERIMENTAL ANIMALS IN THE
QUALITY CONTROL OF VETERINARY VACCINES FOR MAMMALS

Test for freedom from rabies virus	Safety test	Potency test	
			DOG
0	-	±	Hepatitis (i)
0	-	±	Distemper (i)
0	-	±	Leptospirosis (i)
0	-	±	Parvoviral infection (i)
0	-	±	Rabies (i)
+	-	0	Hepatitis (l)
+	-	0	Distemper (l)
+	-	0	Measles (l)
+	-	-	Combined vaccine (l) — **CAT**
0	-	-	Influenza (i) — **HORSE**
0	-	+	Tetanus (t)
0	-	±	Brucella abortis (i) — **CATTLE**
0	-	±	E.coli (i)
0	-	-	Lungworm
0	-	-	Anthrax (i)
0	-	±	Foot-and-mouth dis. (i)
0	-	±	Atrophic rhinitis (i) — **PIG**
0	-		Aujeszky's disease (l)
0	-	±	Cl. perfrigens (t)
0	-	±	E.coli (i)
0	-	-	Influenza (i)
0	-	±	Swine Erysipelas (i)
0	-	±	Aujeszky's disease (i)

i = inactivated; l = live; t = toxoid.
For a key to the symbols see chapter 8, table 1.

In so far that official guidelines exist for this test, it is based on an in vitro method for some products (e.g. equine influenza vaccine), and on an in vivo method for other vaccines (e.g. the clostridial vaccines). The latter involves subcutaneous administration of 0.5 ml of the vaccine to each of 5 mice. The assessment criterion used is the development of local and systemic reactions.

3. VACCINES FOR DOGS

3.1. Potency test on inactivated vaccines
3.1.1. Leptospirosis vaccine
The potency test for the leptospirosis vaccine stipulated by the official guidelines (e.g.in the European Pharmacopoeia) (1) is based on a lethal challenge in hamsters. Until recently, this was the only animal model available for determining the protective action of this vaccine. A positive correlation with the activity of the vaccine in dogs has been demonstrated (2). However, the method has several shortcomings:
- it requires a large number of animals and entails a high degree of distress;
- it is not very reproducible, chiefly because of the problem of standardizing the challenging suspension of virulent leptospirae (these are obtained from the kidneys or spleens of infected hamsters);
- the hamster is difficult to handle;
- the laboratory personnel run a risk of infection.
It has recently been reported that the content of neutralizing antibodies induced by the vaccine can be estimated serologically in the dog (3, 4) by means of an ELISA. Meanwhile, the guinea pig has also been found to be a suitable model for this purpose, and it should now be established whether there is a positive correlation between this serological assay and the protective action of the vaccine in the dog (5). The preliminary results of such a study indicate that its substitution for the lethal challenge procedure in hamsters should be given serious consideration. There is, however, another advantage as far as animal usage is concerned,which will be discussed below.

3.1.2. Canine parvovirus, hepatitis (HCC) and distemper vaccines
Although neither the European Pharmacopoeia nor the British Pharmacopoeia contains guidelines for the potency test on the parvovirus vaccine, manufacturers determine its potency on the basis of the serological response in guinea pigs. In the US Code of Federal Regulations the in vivo test has recently been replaced by an in vitro assay based on haemagglutination (6). It is not yet clear how well this antigenicity determination is correlated with the immunity induced in the dog, and further study is needed to validate it.
Another approach holds better prospects, and consists of combining the potency tests of the inactivated vaccines (except the rabies vaccine) into a single serological test on guinea pigs. Although the potency of the hepatitis and distemper vaccines is still assessed in dogs (also based on serology), the guinea pig can in principle also be used as a model and this is currently being studied. Preliminary results suggest that this approach may be feasible. (4).

3.1.3. Rabies vaccine

The difficulty of replacing the in vivo potency test was
discussed in connection with the human rabies vaccine. This also
applies to the rabies vaccine for veterinary use. In both cases
the determination is based on an intracerebral challenge in mice.
Alternative methods which were discussed for the human rabies
vaccine, such as single radial immunodiffusion (SRD), ELISA and
the antibody binding test (ABT), can in principle also be used in
the potency testing of the veterinary vaccine, but these in vitro
assays are less suitable for testing veterinary rabies vaccines
based on brain tissues, or vaccines containing aluminium
hydroxide as an adjuvant. For the latter category of vaccines a
refinement of the technique could offer a solution, the virus
being first separated from the adjuvant after which the "potency"
(that is the antigenicity) can be estimated in vitro.

3.2. Potency tests on live, attenuated vaccines

As mentioned before, the in vivo potency test is required for
only one representative vaccine batch of a seed lot. An in vitro
determination may be sufficient for the other batches (titration
of the virus in a tissue culture system). This means that the in
vivo potency test is performed only occasionally. Nevertheless,
it can be recommended that here too an effort be made to reduce
and/or refine the use of animals, particularly since the
determination is often based on a lethal challenge test. Table 2
lists the specifications of the existing guidelines for the once-
only potency test on a live vaccine for dogs, in this particular
case the canine distemper vaccine. Species, number of animals and
assessememt criterion are roughly the same for the other dog
vaccines. A striking - and probably unnecessary - feature is the
large number of animals specified by the FDA guidelines.

Table 2: SPECIFICATIONS FOR THE ONCE-ONLY POTENCY TEST ON CANINE
DISTEMPER VACCINE

		Distress category 4*		
Specifications	J	Eur.Ph.(7)	UK (8)	USA (9)
Species	dog	dog	dog	dog
No. of animal groups	1	1	1	1
No. of animals/group	5	7	5	20
Route of administration	i.m.	as per label	as per label	n.s.
Duration:				
- immunization (weeks)	3-4	3	3	3
- observation after challenge (weeks)	3	3	3	3
No. of control groups	1	1	1	1
- no. of dogs/group	2	2	2	5
Mode of challenge	s.o.	s.o./i.c./ i.v.	s.o./i.c. i.v.	i.c.
Criterion		.... death of controls; serology		

```
*     = See chapter 5, section 4
n.s.  = not specified          i.m. = intramuscular;
i.c.  = intracerebral          s.o. = suboccipital;
i.v.  = intravenous;
Note: J refers to a Dutch manufacturer's specifications.
```

3.3. Test for freedom from contaminating rabies virus

The test for freedom from rabies virus is part of the quality
control of the live, attenuated vaccines for cats and dogs. One
or more groups of mice are given an intracerebral, and sometimes
also an intraperitoneal, injection of the vaccine. The animals
should manifest no abnormal reactions during the observation
period. Table 3 lists the existing guidelines' specifications for
this examination.

Table 3: SPECIFICATIONS FOR THE TEST FOR FREEDOM FROM RABIES
         VIRUS

		Distress category 2*		
Specifications	K	Eur.Ph.(10)	UK (8)	USA (9)
Species	mouse	mouse	mouse	mouse
No. of animal groups	1	1	1	2
No. of animals/group	5	5	5	8
Route of administration	i.c.	i.c.	i.c.	i.c./i.p.
Control group	yes,1	no	no	no
- no. of animals/group	5			
Observation period (weeks)	3	3	2	1
Criterion		.... clinical signs and symptoms		

*   = See chapter 5, section 4
i.c. = intracerebral;   i.p. = intraperitoneal.
Note: K refers to the specifications of a Dutch manufacturer.

The absence of rabies virus is one of the safety requirements a
vaccine has to satisfy in order to be accepted for general use.
In the past, this test was certainly not superfluous, but it may
be questioned how relevant it still is today. In the past decade,
in particular, the vaccine production process has been
extensively standardized and validated, partly owing to the
introduction of GMP. In addition, the quality of the animals used
for vaccine production has been greatly improved. The many
precautions taken in the production of vaccines rule out the
likelihood of contamination of a vaccine batch, especially when
the vaccines are made in a laboratory where rabies virus is not
used. A proposal to the European Pharmacopoeia Commission to
discontinue the test for rabies virus, with the provision that
the virus is not used within an establishment for production or
research purposes, would link up with a proposal made recently to
the US Food and Drug Administration (FDA) to change the American
guidelines for this check (11).

4. VACCINES FOR HORSES

4.1. Potency test on influenza vaccine

The value of the single radial immunodiffusion (SRD) technique
was mentioned in the paragraph on the human influenza vaccine.
This in vitro method is based on the reaction of the influenza
haemagglutinin (HA) with a specific anti-HA serum in agarose gel
and is basically an antigenicity determination.
An SRD method has also been developed for the equine influenza
vaccine. A good correlation between the HA concentration and the
content of protective antibodies has been found in field trials

(12). However, application of the _in vitro_ technique is limited to in-process control for the time being, because the veterinary, unlike the human, influenza vaccines are adjuvated products*. Before an SRD determination can be made the adjuvant has to be separated from the virus, which may result in some loss of antigen. Acceptable separation techniques are not yet available and until such a technique has been developed the potency test of the final product must be estimated by an _in vivo_ test.

These _in vivo_ tests are currently based on a serological estimation in horses (one representative vaccine batch from a seed lot) and in guinea pigs (the other batches derived from the same seed lot).

4.2. Potency test on tetanus vaccine

In general the same procedure is employed as for estimating the potency of some other clostridial vaccines, that is, vaccination of guinea pigs, followed by titration of their sera by toxin neutralization in groups of mice.

No real _in vitro_ alternative is available at the moment. However, replacing the above mentioned method by the lethal or paralytic challenge procedure requiring fewer animals (see chapter 8, section 6.3.) would be a first step towards a reduction of animal usage.

5. VACCINES FOR CATTLE

5.1. Potency test on Brucella abortus vaccine

A commonly used procedure to estimate the potency of this vaccine involves two groups of guinea pigs, one group being vaccinated and the other serving as a control. After an immunization period of 6 weeks, the animals are challenged with live Brucella abortus bacteria. Five to 6 weeks after the challenge, culture plates are inoculated with spleen suspension prepared from these animals, which are then assessed on the basis of bacterial growth.

According to a recent publication (14), specific antibodies to Brucella abortus can be detected in cattle by the ELISA technique, using purified antigen. Although no research has yet been carried out into the possible application of this method in vaccine quality control, it could serve as a starting point for a serological approach to potency testing.

5.2. Potency test on footh-and-mouth disease vaccine

Foot-and-mouth disease is the single most important disease of cattle. Since the development of an inactivated vaccine, animals are immunized in many countries against this disease.

Most control authorities stipulate determination of the PD50 (median protective dose) in cattle as a potency test. Serial five-fold dilutions of the vaccine are inoculated into groups of from 5 to 8 animals, each group receiving one dilution, and 2 animals serve as controls.

The animals are injected intradermally with the virulent challenge virus into the tongue 21 days after vaccination.

---

* It was actually claimed by Wood (13) that the SRD assay is not affected by the presence of an adjuvant in the vaccine. Further study has shown that the type of adjuvant determines whether or not it is possible to carry out the potency test _in vitro_ using the SRD method.

The potency with 95% fudicial limits is calculated statistically
on the basis of the manifestations of secondary lesions in their
feet, these being a sign of incomplete protection against foot-
and-mouth disease. Table 4 summarizes the guidelines and their
specifications for the potency testing of foot-and-mouth disease
vaccine.

Table 4: THE SPECIFICATIONS OF EXISTING GUIDELINES FOR THE
POTENCY TEST ON FOOT-AND-MOUTH DISEASE VACCINE

| Specifications | Distress category 4* | | |
	Neth. (15)	Eur.Ph.(16)	UK (17)
Species	cattle	cattle	cattle
No. of animal groups	n.s.	n.s.	3
No. of animals/group	5	≥ 5	5
Control group	1	1	1
- no. of animals/group	2	2	2
Duration:			
- immunization (weeks)	3	3	3
- observation after			
challenge (days)	8	8	8
Mode of challenge	i.d.	i.d.	i.d.
	tongue	tongue	tongue
Criterion	... lesions in tongue and feet ...		

* see chapter 5, section 4.
n.s. = not specified;   i.d. = intradermal.

There are several disadvantages attached to this challenge
evaluation (18):
- the method causes considerable pain and distress and involves
  some risk, due to the use of virulent virus;
- only one serotype can be evaluated per experiment, so that the
  method is commercially unattractive;
- a quantitative assay based on a relatively small number of
  animals is very inaccurate (the 90% confidence interval for the
  PD50 value lies between 45% and 220% of the potency).

In spite of these drawbacks no in vitro assay system is yet
available, and using small laboratory animals for potency testing
has also proved impossible.
An approach removing a few of the negative aspects of the PD50
determination was described a few years ago (19, 20), and is
based on the determination of the serum antibody titre in
vaccinated animals. Validation on 38 vaccine batches indicated
that there is a good correlation between the logarithm of the
serum antibody titres (log SNT) and the PD50 values (19). This
makes it possible to estimate the potency of vaccine batches by a
serum antibody assay. It was pointed out in the same article that
any mutation of the vaccine virus makes it necessary to establish
this correlation anew for which a new PD50 determination must be
made.

5.3. Safety test on foot-and-mouth disease vaccine

The safety test on the foot-and-mouth disease vaccine is aimed chiefly at the presence of non-inactivated virus. The European Pharmacopoeia guidelines for this test specify an intradermal injection of the vaccine into the tongues of cattle, this being the most sensitive method. In vitro procedures have been proposed. However, adsorption of the vaccine virus precedes its inactivation during the production process, and the presence of the adsorbent interferes with the cell culture. On the other hand, it is now possible to separate the vaccine virus from the adsorbent after its inactivation and to evaluate the resulting concentrate in cell cultures. In this connection, cultures of foetal calf thyroid gland cells (21) and baby hamster kidney (BHK) cells (22) have already been described.

The in vitro model is a sensitive method for demonstrating the presence of incompletely inactivated virus, in part because - unlike the in vivo method - large amounts of inactivated virus do not interfere with the detection of virulent virus. Nevertheless, it is not yet possible to dispense with the in vivo test for safety considerations, and both methods must be employed in the quality control.

5.4. Potency test on E.coli vaccine

The design and execution of the potency test on the bovine and on the swine E.coli vaccines are the same, and discussed in more detail in section 6.3.

6. VACCINES FOR PIGS

6.1. Potency test on clostridial vaccines

The statutory test for estimating the potency of Clostridium perfringens vaccine, but also for a number of other veterinary clostridial vaccines (Cl. septicum, Cl. novyi), is based on indirect toxin neutralization in mice (23). Rabbits are first immunized with the vaccine being tested, and the antibodies produced in response to it are assayed by toxin neutralization in mice. This protocol involves fairly large numbers of animals; the testing requirements of the Dutch manufacturers of veterinary vaccines specify about 4 rabbits and 50 mice per batch.

The potency test of the Clostridium perfringens vaccine is estimated as specified by the European Pharmacopoeia guideline (23). At least 10 rabbits are immunized twice with the vaccine being tested and exsanguinated after an immunization period of 31 to 42 days. The strength of the pooled sera is determined in a suitable laboratory species, usually the mouse. Dilutions of the pooled serum under examination or of a standard antitoxin are incubated with constant amounts of Clostridium perfringens toxin. Of each mixture, 0.5 ml is injected either intravenously or intraperitoneally into groups of at least 2 mice. The assessment criterion used is death of the animals within 72 hours. The experiment is repeated at least once and the mean strenght of the serum is calculated in relation to the standard antitoxin used. The strength of the serum is a measure of the efficacy of the vaccine.

In general, a similar procedure is followed in the potency testing of the Cl. septicum and Cl. novyi vaccines.

For the Cl. chauvoei (24) and Cl. botulinum (25) vaccines, the potency assay is based on a qualitative lethal challenge test in guinea pigs and a qualitative paralytic challenge test in mice, respectively.

Research into the possibility of estimating antigenicity by in
vitro methods (20) showed that there is no correlation between
the amount of vaccine antigen found in the in vitro assay and the
degree of immunity produced in the animal. Consequently, genuine
in vitro assays do not appear feasible for the time being.
However, there are several other possibilities which may make the
toxin neutralization in mice unnecessary. One possibility is to
immunize rabbits and then to determine the antibody titre by an
immunological in vitro technique. Consistent and reproducible
results were obtained with the Cl. perfringens vaccine, using the
technique of immunoelectrophoresis, and validation showed a good
correlation between this and the in vivo method. Unfortunately,
the results were less consistent with the Cl. septicum and Cl.
novyi vaccines. It has been reported that in this case prior
purification of the reagents used (e.g. the toxoid) may provide
the solution (26).
Not yet studied but possibly applicable is the recently described
in vitro model for determining the titre of tetanus antibodies in
human sera (27). Translated to the veterinary clostridial
vaccines this would amount to immunization and exsanguination in
rabbits, followed by an in vitro determination of the antibody
titre. The procedure involves incubating dilutions of the serum
with constant amounts of toxin. Next, any free toxin present is
demonstrated with the help of an antibody-coated ELISA plate.
Another approach is based on toxin neutralization in cell
cultures, (e.g. Vero cells). To study the feasibility of this
approach, experiments with 3 types of Clostridium vaccine have
been carried out. It was found that the antibody titre determined
by the in vitro method was generally lower than that measured
with the in vivo techniques. Thus, the correlation with the
animal test found for the Cl. septicum vaccine was good, but it
was much less favourable for the Cl. novyi and Cl. perfringens
vaccines (28). It may be concluded that, in general, the
potential of in vitro neutralization techniques for reducing the
number of animals used in the potency testing of these vaccines
is great, but further improvement and validation of these methods
are still necessary.

6.2. Potency test on swine influenza vaccine
The remarks made about the possibility of alternative methods for
the potency testing of equine influenza vaccine (chapter 11,
section 4.1.) also apply here.

6.3. Potency test on vaccines against atrophic rhinitis, E. coli
infection and swine erysipelas
The potency test on these vaccines is based on the same general
principle: groups of mice are immunized and then challenged with
the virulent agent. There are two approaches: the first consists
of using several vaccine dilutions and one challenging dose, the
second of using one vaccine dilution and several challenging
doses. One or more control groups are also included. The
assessment criterion used is lethality. Official guidelines exist
only for the potency test on swine erysipelas vaccine, the
details of which are given in table 5.
The specifications for the pig vaccines are for the most part
based on data and results obtained during the development stage.
However, as the production of a vaccine proceeds with time, our
knowledge, and therefore also the standardizability, of the
potency test may be expected to increase through its routine
application. As a result, the number of animals originally used

134

for this test is no longer necessary for routine quality control
and could thus be reduced. However, the test requirements of the
various guidelines do not permit this. It could be recommended
therefore to re-evaluate and adapt the specifications on the
basis of the experience gained with the routine control over a
period of, say, 2 years after a product has been submitted for
registration. This general recommendation could also be made for
the potency testing of pig vaccines. There are indications that
the large number of animals currently used could be reduced (29).
It may be useful to carry out the same evaluation of the potency
test here as that made for the diphtheria and tetanus vaccine,
i.e., to determine on the basis of previously conducted research,
using computer models, the effect of a reduction in group size on
the outcome of the test.

Table 5: SPECIFICATIONS OF THE EXISTING GUIDELINES FOR THE
POTENCY TEST ON SWINE ERYSIPELAS VACCINE

Specifications	Distress category*		
	Eur.Ph.(29)	UK (17)	USA (9)
Species	mouse	mouse	mouse
No. of animal groups	3	3	3
No. of animals/group	16	10	16
Route of administration	s.c.	s.c.	s.c.
Reference vaccine	yes	yes	yes
- no. of animal groups	3	3	3
- no. of animals/group	16	10	16
Duration:			
- immunization (days)	21	21	14-21
- observation after challenge (days)	8	8	10
No. of control groups	1	1	n.s.
- no. of animals/group	10	10	
Mode of challenge	i.p.	i.p.	n.s.
Criterion	.... death		

* See chapter 5, section 4.
s.c. = subcutaneous;   i.p. = intraperitoneal;
n.s. = not specified

7. SUMMARY

The following recommendations can be made for reducing or
refining the use of experimental animals in the quality control
of vaccines for mammals.

7.1. Dogs
INACTIVATED VACCINES
- Leptospirosis vaccine:
  - potency test: - replacement of the lethal challenge procedure
                    in hamsters by a serological estimation in
                    guinea pigs.

- Leptospirosis, parvovirus infection, hepatitis and distemper vaccines:
  - potency test: - combination of the various assays into a single potency test based on a serological assessment in guinea pigs.

- Rabies vaccine:
  - potency test: - validation of the ELISA or antibody binding test (ABT) (see the human rabies vaccine).

LIVE, ATTENUATED VACCINES
- Hepatitis, distemper and measles vaccines:
  - test for contamination with rabies virus:
            - discontinuation of this test subject to the conditions mentioned under section 3.3.

7.2. Cat
- Live combined vaccine:
  - test for contamination with rabies virus:
            - discontinuation of this test subject to the conditions mentioned under section 3.3.

7.3. Horse
- tetanus vaccine:
  - potency test: - replacement of the indirect toxinneutralization assay on guinea pigs and mice by the lethal or paralytic challenge test in mice, and reduction of the number of animals per group as for the human tetanus vaccine.

7.4. Cattle
- Brucella abortus vaccine:
  - potency test: - examination of the possible replacement of the challenge test by a serological estimation.

- Foot-and-mouth disease vaccine:
  - potency test: - validation of an alternative approach based on serology to replace the challenge test.
  - safety test: - validation of an in vitro model using foetal calf thyroid gland cells or baby hamster kidney cells.

- E. coli vaccine:
  - potency test: - examination of possible reduction in the number of animals used per vaccine dilution.

7.5. Pig
- Clostridial vaccines:
  - potency test: - validation of several in vitro toxin neutralization models to replace the lethal challenge test in mice.

- Atrophic rhinitis, swine erysipelas, E. coli and inactivated Aujeszky vaccines:
  - potency test: - examination of possible reduction in the number of animals used per vaccine dilution.

8. REFERENCES

1. European Pharmacopoeia, Mon. 447 (1985)
2. Huhn, R.G. et al.: Immunity to leptospirosis: bacterins in dogs and hamsters. Am. J. Vet. Res. (1975), 36, 1, 71-74
3. Hartman, E.G. et al.: Serodiagnosis of canine leptospirosis by solid-phase enzyme-linked immunosorbent assay. Vet. Immunology and Immunopathology, (1984), 7, 33-42
4. Hartman, E.G. et al.: Determination of specific anti-leptospiral immunoglobulins M and G of experimentally infected dogs by solid-phase enzyme-linked immunosorbent assay. Vet. Immunology and Immunopathology, (1984), 7, 43-51
5. Pereboom W.J.: Personal communication
6. Hyde, R.L.W.: Reduction of in vivo testing at the National Veterinary Services Laboratories of the United States Department of Agriculture. Develop. Biol. Standard. (1986), 64, 149-151
7. European Pharmacopoeia, Mon. 451 (1985)
8. British Pharmacopoeia (Vet.), 1985
9. Code of Federal Regulations, (1984), 9, FDA
10. European Pharmacopoeia, Vol. III, Suppl. (1977)
11. Federal Register (FDA), Vol. 49, 112, 23864, (1984)
12. Wood, J.M. et al.: Single-radial-immunodiffusion potency tests of inactivated influenza vaccines for use in man and animals. Develop. Biol. Standard. (1986), 64, 169-177
13. Wood, J.M. et al.: The standardization of inactivated equine influenza vaccines by single radial immunodiffusion. Journ. Biol. Standard. (1983), 11, 133-136
14. Tabatabai, L.B. and Deyoe, B.L.: Specific enzyme-linked immunosorbent assay for detection of bovine antibody to Brucella abortus. Jour. Clinical Microbiology (1984), 20, 2, 209-213
15. Nederlandse Farmacopee (Dutch Pharmacopoeia), Vol. 2, 9th edition, (1983)
16. European Pharmacopoeia, Mon. 63 (1985)
17. British Pharmacopoeia (Vet.), (1977)
18. Pay, T.W.F. and Hingley, P.J.: The use of serum neutralizing antibody assay for the determination of the potency of foot-and-mouth disease (FMD) vaccines in cattle. Develop. Biol. Standard. (1986), 64, 153-161
19. Pay, T.W.F. and Parker, M.J.: Some statistical and experimental design problems in the assessment of FMD vaccine potency. Develop. Biol. Standard. (1977), 35, 369-383
20. Hingley, P.J. and Pay, T.W.F.: Sources of variability in foot-and-mouth disease vaccine potency estimates based on serum neutralizing antibody assay. Jour. Biol. Standard. (1987), 15, 127-143
21. Barteling, S.J. et al.: Innocuity of foot-and-mouth disease vaccines. I. Formaldehyde-inactivated alhydrogel vaccines. Jour. Biol. Standard. (1983), 11, 297-304
22. Anderson, E.C. et al.: In vitro method for safety testing of foot-and-mouth disease vaccines. J. Hyg. Camb. (1970), 68, 159-172
23. European Pharmacopoeia, Mon. 363, (1984)
24. European Pharmacopoeia, Mon. 361, (1984)
25. European Pharmacopoeia, Mon. 360, (1984)
26. White, V.J. and Sojka, M.G.: Immunoelectrophoresis in quality control of veterinary clostridial products. Develop. Biol. Standard. (1986), 64, 119-127

27. Hendriksen, C.F.M. et al.: The toxin binding inhibition test as a reliable in vitro alternative to the toxin neutralization test in mice for the estimation of tetanus antitoxin in human sera. Jour. Biol. Standard. (1988), 16, 4, (In press)

28. Knight, P.A. et al.: The titration of clostridial toxoids and antisera in cell culture. Develop. Biol. Standard. (1986), 64, 129-136

29. Pereboom, W.J.: Personal communication

CHAPTER 12: REPLACEMENT, REDUCTION OR REFINEMENT: AN INDIRECT
APPROACH

1. INTRODUCTION

Several proposals and recommendations were made in the previous
chapters with regard to the reduction or refinement of the use of
animals for specific tests in the quality control of vaccines.
These proposals generally implied a more or less drastic change
in the relevant animal test.
However, a reduction in animal usage may also be achievable
through an indirect approach: it may be possible to reduce the
number of laboratory animals or animal tests, or the pain and
distress caused, by changing the conditions under which a
particular animal test is performed.
The following ways towards achieving this goal will be discussed
briefly:
- harmonizing the guidelines;
- reviewing the need for re-testing by the national control
  laboratories;
- combining several tests;
- using inbred animal strains;
- increasing the size of vaccine batches;
- relaxing the body weight specifications;
- re-using animals;
- using specific pathogen-free (SPF) animals;
- reducing or suppressing pain.

2. HARMONIZING THE GUIDELINES

The animal experiments performed in the quality control of
vaccines are subject to strict regulation. The test
specifications of the existing guidelines may differ as regards
numbers of animals, numbers of animal groups, modes of
administration, methodologies, etc. As a result, when a product
is submitted to the regulatory authorities in several countries
for registration, the total number of animal tests required for
this particular product may be greater than the number stipulated
by each of the individual countries.
In some instances these differences in guidelines rest on a well-
founded necessity, but in other cases they are based on marketing
rather than on scientific grounds, and at least a proportion of
the animals used is determined by politics. Since export
interests are an important factor in veterinary vaccine
production, the above-mentioned problems are most evident with
this category of vaccines.
All this underlines the need for international harmonization of
the various guidelines. Its realization could make an important
contribution to the effort to reduce the use of experimental
animals. The European Pharmacopoeia Commission is doing
invaluable work in this field through the publication of its
monographs, which have the status of official guidelines for the
participating Western European countries.
Nevertheless, they still allow the individual member states to
deviate from the European guidelines. Many of the monographs
contain the clause: "..... Subject to agreement by the national
control authority", thereby leaving open the possibility of
adopting divergent guidelines.

The guidelines formulated by the WHO, and published in the
Technical Report Series, could contribute significantly to
supranational harmonization. However, they have no official
status but are only recommendations, and it is left to each
national control authority to make them legally binding. While
the development of alternative methods is a contribution from the
scientific community towards the reduction of animal usage, it is
especially in the field of international cooperation that
governments and other policy-making bodies can contribute towards
this goal. It is ultimately the governments of the various member
states which are responsible for the policy embodied in, for
example, the European Pharmacopoeia, and thus for the extent of
harmonization of their guidelines.
The recognition in one country of the results of animal tests
obtained in another in order to avoid unnecessary duplication of
tests lies in the same political sphere. For example, a vaccine
that has been submitted for registration to the national control
authority in different countries may undergo animal testing more
than once. The Convention drawn up by the Council of Europe for
the protection of laboratory animals includes an article
concerning the mutual recognition of animal test results (1).
However, the wording of this article is such that it allows each
of the member states considerable leeway. It can be recommended
that an effort be made to achieve complete harmonization of the
guidelines and requirements on a European level, which could only
be deviated from after a critical examination of the arguments by
a Community arbitration committee.
An even more intricate task is to achieve harmonization and
cooperation on a supranational level. Although this can only be
formulated in general terms, it should be stressed that both
harmonization and cooperation are a prerequisite for an effective
approach to the 3 Rs concept.

3. REVIEWING THE NEED FOR RE-TESTING BY THE NATIONAL CONTROL AUTHORITIES

In most countries there is an agency which, completely
independent of the vaccine producers and quality controllers,
ultimately decides on the release of a batch of vaccine for
general use. This is the National Control Authority. It arrives
at its decision after checking the production and quality control
data against the existing guidelines or regulations. Where
necessary, it verifies the data by research in its own
laboratories, which in some cases involves repeating the relevant
animal tests. This re-testing is in principle understandable in
view of the fact that the national control authority is
ultimately responsible for the release of a vaccine for general
use. However, vaccine production and control are increasingly
determined by the rules of GMP which require, among other things,
the keeping of records of production and quality control data,
and validation of the production process and quality control
tests, all under the supervision of an independent body.
Automation also contributes to the standardization of production
and control.
Viewed in this light, it seems sensible to review the need for
re-testing by the national control authorities. It will not be
feasible to discontinue it in all cases but opportunities do
exist, which depend on the type of product and the extent to
which the GMP rules have been implemented within a production and
control establishment.

4. COMBINING SEVERAL TESTS

The possibility of combining several tests was explored in the chapters on human bacterial vaccines and poultry and dog vaccines. Another opportunity exists with those potency tests in which a standard preparation is also included. One standard-vaccine determination only is sufficient if several batches of the same vaccine type are evaluated simultaneously for their potency. A prerequisite for this is that the assays are made under the same conditions, that is, in the same room and at the same time.

5. USING INBRED ANIMAL STRAINS

Random-bred strains of laboratory animals are normally used in the quality control of vaccines and only rarely are inbred strains used for this purpose. It is known that the former do not have a uniform reaction pattern (see also chapter 3). The greater uniformity of an inbred strain means that fewer animals are needed for a test to achieve the same degree of statistical precision. However, there are unfortunately some differences in sensitivity between inbred strains, so that their introduction into the quality control of vaccines would entail that for each animal test a specifically sensitive strain would have to be found (2). This is difficult to achieve for both practical and scientific reasons.
Furthermore, the reaction pattern of inbred strains is particularly sensitive to external influences. These drawbacks can be eliminated by choosing either the factorial design - in which animals are divided into a number of subgroups of different inbred strains - or Fl hybrids, i.e. the first filial generation produced by crossing two inbred strains, instead of the latter themselves.
No information exists about the practicability of the factorial design or of Fl hybrids, and their possible impact on the total number of animals required. Because of the fairly small size of the animal groups used in the quality control of vaccines (unlike with certain tests in toxicology), introduction of the factorial design is not feasible.However, an exploratory study or a cost-benefit analysis of the use of Fl hybrids does merit consideration.

6. INCREASING THE SIZE OF VACCINE BATCHES

Recent improvements in the production process have made it possible to prepare homogeneous vaccine batches in relatively large volumes (up to 1000 litres). Since the extent of quality control depends more on the number of batches to be tested than on the size of a single batch, increasing the batch volume will reduce the number of tests to be performed, e.g. for potency. However, the possibility of increasing batch volume is limited by the technical difficulties arising in the culturing of large volumes of vaccine bacteria or viruses. It is conceivable that novel production techniques (see chapter 13) could provide the solution to this problem in the future.
The effect of increasing the capacity of the packaging equipment on the frequency of the abnormal-toxicity test has already been mentioned in chapter 8, section 2.3. It seems likely that tangible results can be expected in this field in the near future.

7. RELAXING THE BODY WEIGHT SPECIFICATIONS

The various national and international guidelines specify not
only the species and number of experimental animals to be used
but also their body weight at the start of the test, which must
often be within a certain range. This weight requirement can
hamper the efficient use of experimental animals in two ways.
Firstly, it complicates the planning of breeding programmes and,
secondly, a proportion of the animals (often over 10% of the
stock) fails to meet the weight requirement and must be killed
because there is no further use for them. Table 1 summarizes the
weight requirements of the national and international guidelines
for a few of the human bacterial vaccines discussed in chapter 8.

Table 1: REQUIRED WEIGHTS (IN GRAMS) OF EXPERIMENTAL ANIMALS FOR
VACCINE TESTING

Vaccine test	species	Neth.	WHO	Eur.Ph.	USA	Japan
Tetanus potency	mouse	10- 14	14- 20	17- 22	-	-
Tetanus potency	g.p.	-	250-350	250-350	450-550	300-400
Tetanus abn.tox.	g.p.	350	250-350	250-350	400	±350
	mouse	17- 22	17- 22	-	22	-
Tetanus spec.tox.	g.p.	230-350	250-350	250-350	-	300-400
Diphth. potency	g.p.	250-350	250-350	250-350	450-550	300-400
Diphth. abn.tox.	g.p.	350	250-350	250-350	400	±350
	mouse	17- 22	17- 22	-	22	-
Diphth. spec.tox.	g.p.	250-350	250-350	250-350	-	300-400
Pert. potency	mouse	10- 14	10- 18	Diff. animals 5	10- 20	-
Pert. w-g test	mouse	14- 17	14- 16	-	14- 16	-
BCG	J. test	g.p.	400-500		350	250
BCG	f-f-M.Tub.	g.p.	250-350	250-350	400	250-350	-

g.p.	= guinea pig;	abn.tox.	= abnormal toxicity
Diphth.	= Diphtheria;	spec.tox.	= specific toxicity
Pert.	= Pertussis;	w-g test	= weight-gain test;
f-f-M.Tub.	= freedom from M.tuberc.;	J. test	= Jensen test;
Diff.	= Weight difference between.		

It shows that the weight requirements differ markedly, with the
exception of the tests where weight gain is used as the
assessment criterion (mouse-weight-gain test and abnormal-
toxicity test). It is obvious that the weights of the animals
should not differ too much for the test to be statistically
reliable, but the relevance of rigid weight requirements should
also be examined (this does not apply to the tests in which
young, growing animals are used, such as in the mouse-weight-gain
test). A proposal could be made to relax the weight
specifications by merely stating the range within which the
weight of the animals is allowed to vary without stipulating
their actual weights. This would have definitive advantages for
the planning of the supply of laboratory animals and thus for a
more efficient use of these animals. Since tests must be
reproducible, this proposal can be put into practice in the

potency test only when a standard preparation is also included in it.

8. RE-USING ANIMALS

For a number of quality control tests the experimental procedure need not necessarily result in the death of the animals, and the surviving animals need not always be sacrificed. These animals could be re-used for further tests provided that they have not been subjected to prolonged distress in the previous experiment. Both the ethical and scientific aspects of re-use should be taken into account. Since criteria - other than personal ones - for re-use are lacking and discussions often deal with generalities, this topic merits further study.

9. USING SPECIFIC PATHOGEN-FREE (SPF) ANIMALS

For the majority of animal tests performed in the quality control of vaccines, regulations exist stating how many animals are allowed to die during the experiment from causes other than the vaccine. If the death rate is too high then the test must often be repeated so that overall animal usage increases. It will be clear that improving the quality of both the experimental animals and the conditions under which they are kept can be recommended both from a scientific point of view and for animal-ethical reasons. The use of SPF animals is a useful step in this direction.

10. REDUCING OR SUPPRESSING PAIN

Despite the recommendations made in this report, the experimental animal will continue to have a function in the quality control of vaccines, sometimes in experiments which entail much pain and distress for the animals involved. It is important that this be given serious thought. Since figures speak plainly, there is often greater interest in the replacement and reduction of animal use than in the refinement of experimental procedures, yet this last aspect also deserves special attention.
In the last few years in particular, methods have been developed which reduce or suppress pain in experimental animals (3). On the initiative of the British Pharmacopoeia Commission, the possible use of the analgesic buprenorphine in the potency test of the Clostridium chauvoei vaccine in guinea pigs has recently been studied. But no clear opinion could be given on the basis of the results obtained (4) about the value of buprenorphine. However, it was found that this analgesic did not interfere with the potency test itself.
The subject of pain and distress in small laboratory animals still lies in the twilight zone of science and is governed all too frequently by subjective assessment criteria. This impairs the effective prevention or combatting of pain and distress. Objective criteria to assess these aspects of animal usage have recently been described (5), but they need further elaboration before they can be used as a corollary to any proposal for reducing the degree of distress inflicted upon experimental animals in a test.

11. REFERENCES

1. Council of Europe: European Convention for the protection of vertebrate animals used for experimental and other scientific purposes. Strassbourg, 18 March 1986
2. Festing, M.F.W.: The choice of animals in toxicological screening: inbred strains and the factorial design of experiment. Acta Zool. Pathol. Antwerp. (1980), 75, 117-131
3. Flecknell, P.A.: The relief of pain in laboratory animals. Laboratory Animals (1984), 18, 147-160
4. Council of Europe: Use of experimental animals. Communication from the British Pharmacopoeia Commission. Strassbourgh, 17 July 1987
5. Morton, D.B. and Griffiths, P.H.M.: Guidelines on the recognition of pain, distress and discomfort in experimental animals and on hypothesis for assessment. The Veterinary Record (1985), 116, 431-436

CHAPTER 13: FUTURE PROSPECTS

1. INTRODUCTION

The emphasis in human medicine is gradually shifting from cure to
prevention, as exemplified by the advantages being made in
immunoprophylaxis. After the establishment of a basic vaccination
programme for the entire population, the focus is now on
combatting infectious diseases which occur in specific groups of
the population as well as on developing vaccines against tropical
protozoal diseases. Recent successes in this field include the
vaccines against hepatitis B, malaria and meningococcal
infections. In addition, efforts are being made to intensify
vaccination campaigns in the developing countries through the
"Expanded Programme on Immunization" of the WHO. Similar
developments are under way in veterinary medicine, where vaccines
against parasitic diseases are now generating considerable.
interest.
Since all the areas mentioned involve animal experimentation, the
global use of experimental animals for the production and control
of immunological products will, quite apart from the
recommendations made in this report, show a tendency to rise
rather than fall. This is sufficient reason in itself to take the
recommendations made here seriously. Nevertheless, a certain
optimism is justified as regards the future use of animals in the
vaccine field, because progress is being made in both the
production and control of vaccines, as outlined in the following
paragraphs.

2. VACCINE PRODUCTION

The value of conventional vaccine production as described in
chapter 4 is beyond doubt. Nevertheless, it suffers from several
drawbacks (1, 2):
- attenuated vaccine strains can mutate resulting in an increase
  in virulence or loss of immunogenicity;
- with inactivated vaccines, there is a risk of incomplete
  inactivation;
- it is sometimes difficult to separate toxic components from the
  vaccine microorganisms, so that vaccination may be accompanied
  by adverse reactions (e.g. with the whole-cell pertussis
  vaccine);
- certain microorganisms, such as the hepatitis B virus, cannot
  be cultured by conventional techniques;
- the substrate used for production of viral vaccines in
  particular is a potential reservoir of contaminating
  microorganisms;
- working with pathogenic vaccine strains carries a health risk;
- the cost of assuring the quality of the current vaccines is
  high.
It is in part because of these shortcomings that other production
techniques are being researched, often utilizing the latest
advances from immunology, molecular biology and biochemistry. For
example, the antigens of a microorganism can now be isolated with
the help of monoclonal antibodies, so that it then becomes
possible to identify and purify the antigens responsible for the
immunity by selective neutralization. In addition, recombinant
DNA techniques can be employed to gain an insight into the

genetic material underlying antigen expression. Biochemical
research has in many instances advanced our knowledge of the
structure of antigens.
With this fundamental knowledge, a rational approach is now being
taken to devise novel vaccine production strategies (which was
not possible with the first vaccines), with most attention being
focused on the following types of vaccine:
- subunit vaccines, produced by isolating the immunogenic
  components using conventional biochemical purification
  techniques;
- subunit vaccines, produced by recombinant DNA technology;
- synthetic peptide vaccines;
- idiotype vaccines, in which anti-idiotype antibodies act as
  antigens.

2.1. Subunit vaccines
The subunit vaccines produced by conventional biochemical
purification methods seem to hold the most promise for the near
future. A recent example is the subunit pertussis vaccine, which
contains the antigenic components LPF (lymphocyte promoting
factor) and FHA (filamentous haemagglutinin). Its efficacy was
recently being tested in a field trial in Sweden.
The advances made in biotechnology have recently focused
attention on the possibility of making recombinant DNA vaccines
in which genetic information for antigen expression is inserted
into alien host systems such as bacteria, yeasts or animal cells
(3, 4). The initial euphoria about the possible applications of
this technology has died down to cautious optimism. It is to be
hoped that the lack of fundamental immunological knowledge and
the problems arising with the purification of the subunits are
only temporary stumbling blocks to a definitive breakthrough (5).
Only a few vaccines produced by recombinant DNA technology are
available at present, e.g., a veterinary E. coli vaccine (6) and
a hepatitis B vaccine (7, 8).

2.2. Synthetic peptide vaccines
Advances in biochemistry have increased the interest in
polypeptide vaccines produced by chemical sythesis. The appeal of
this approach is that it permits the manufacture of chemically
well-defined products on an industrial scale (1). However, it has
meanwhile become clear that, though the required antigenic
peptides can be synthesized, it is very difficult to obtain the
spatial configuration of the peptide chains necessary for
immunogenicity (9). To date, not one peptide vaccine has reached
the stage of clinical trials, and only research on a foot-and-
mouth disease vaccine is in an advanced stage (1).

2.3. Idiotype vaccines
A novel approach to the problem of vaccine production is found
with the so-called (anti-)idiotype vaccines where anti-idiotype
antibodies act as replacements for the antigens. Although the
idea is promising, extensive experimental research is still
needed before it can be applied in practice (10).
The production techniques outlined above can help to reduce the
use of animals in two ways. Firstly, they dispense with animals
for production purposes (though the recombinant DNA vaccines,
based on expression in animal cells, form an exception to this).
Secondly, it is generally believed that these techniques have a
greater potential than the conventional methods for preparing
vaccines that are immunogenically better defined, contain fewer

toxic components, are less liable to contamination and can be made in larger batches. This improvement in quality and quantity will not obviate the need for batch testing but it can reduce its extent and intensity.

Unfortunately, however, novel production technologies have as yet achieved only limited application; they are economically unattractive for producing a number of the conventional vaccines. In addition, production techniques such as recombinant DNA are new phenomena in quality control so that the control authorities tend to be rather cautious in their risk assessment, and add more tests to the quality control instead of abolishing superfluous tests. Consequently, the effect of these new production technologies on animal usage must be viewed with some reserve.

3. VACCINE CONTROL

Whereas the new generation of vaccine production techniques should still be very cautiously observed, a more definite statement can be made about the effect of progress in vaccine control on animal usage. There is a clear tendency here towards reduction and refinement as reflected in, for example, the attempt to adapt and harmonize the guidelines for the quality control tests. However, the developments in the field of alternative methods are of a more structural nature. These have already been discussed in chapters 8-11 for the individual vaccines so that they will here be only briefly outlined.

3.1. Safety evaluation

In vitro techniques are being or can be developed for those animal-based tests which have to answer well-defined questions, such as the test for specific toxicity or the test for specified microorganisms (e.g. the test for residual live virus). In general, the technical and theoretical knowledge already exists so that the emphasis should be on validation of applicable in vitro techniques. The above does not apply to animal tests which are of a general nature such as the test for abnormal toxicity. The replacement of in vivo by in vitro models does not seem feasible here because these tests require that the organs and tissues are in their normal physiological relationship. However, this does not mean that a 3Rs approach is not possible here. As has already been discussed, a reduction in the numbers of animals used can be achieved through an indirect approach, for example, increasing the size of vaccine batches.

3.2. Potency testing

The development of in vitro models for the potency testing of inactivated vaccines will generally occur in two phases. Phase 1 consists of the replacement of the challenge procedure by an in vitro determination of the content of neutralizing antibodies using tissue culture systems or immunological techniques. This development means that the experimental animal will benefit in two ways. First, the distress-causing challenge is replaced by taking blood samples, which causes less suffering. Second, the number of animals required can usually be reduced, because a serum determination is a more accurate assessment criterion than a challenge test. This line of approach has already become feasible (table 1), though it is not always put into effect, for the diphtheria, leptospirosis and clostridial vaccines discussed in the previous chapters.

In phase 2, which is still in the experimental stage, the in
vitro induction of antibody response in, for example, sensitized
human peripheral blood lymphocytes, by an antigen is studied. The
preliminary results of experiments with the tetanus, rabies,
diphtheria and the polio antigens using this technique (11-14)
are so promising that further experimentation and validation can
be highly recommended.
Although the in vitro tests described here concern the
inactivated vaccines in general, their applicability has to be
examined for each type of vaccine, and this is heavily dependent
on the existing fundamental knowledge of the particular vaccine.
But if the outcome is favourable, the opportunity arises to carry
out the potency testing of vaccines entirely in vitro, based on
the methods to be developed in phases 1 and 2.

Table 1. DEVELOPMENT OF ALTERNATIVES WITHIN THE POTENCY TESTING
OF INACTIVATED HUMAN VACCINES

Stage of the potency test	Original procedure	Alternative approach	State of affairs
A. immunization	in vivo immunization	in vitro stimulation of lymphocytes	
		* diphtheria	under dev.
		* tetanus	under dev.
		* pertussis	under dev.
		* polio	under dev.
B. challenge	lethal challenge		
	* diphtheria	serum titration in Vero cells	realized
	* tetanus	serum titration using ELISA	under dev.
	* pertussis	serum titration using ELISA	realized
	* polio	serum titration in Vero cells	realized

under dev. = under development

4. REFERENCES

1. Lerner, R.A.: Synthetic vaccines. Sci. American (1983), 248, 48-56
2. Steward, M.W. and Howard, C.R.: The potential of synthetic peptides for vaccines. Medical Laboratory Sciences, (1985), 42, 376-387
3. Liew, F.Y.: New aspects of vaccine development. Clin. Exp. Immunol. (1985), 62, 225-241
4. Davies, J.E.: Genetic engineering and vaccines. Ann. Inst. Pasteur/Immunol. (1985), 136D, 143-150
5. Korevaar, R.: Biotechnologische vaccins tegen grillige ziekteverwekkers. (Biotechnological vaccines against erratic pathogens.) Toegepaste Wetenschap T.N.O. (1985), 6, 24-29
6. Storm, P.K.: Veterinaire vaccins op basis van recombinant DNA. (Veterinary vaccines based on recombinant DNA.) Tijdschr. Diergeneeskd. (1983), 108, 3, 109-111
7. Smith, G.L. et al.: Infectious vaccinia virus recombinants that express hepatitis B virus surface antigen. Nature (1983), 302, 490-495
8. Anonymous: The production of hepatitis B vaccines in yeast. WHO-Chronicle, (1984), 38, 6, 260-261
9. Ruitenberg, E.J. and Wezel, A.L. van: Biotechnologie en vaccinbereiding. (Biotechnology and vaccine production.) Tijdschr. Diergeneeskd. (1984), 109, 20, 819-821
10. Bona, C. and Moran, T.: Idiotype vaccines. Ann. Inst. Pasteur/Immunol. (1985), 136C, 3, 299-312
11. Kreeftenberg, J.G. et al.: Investigations on the immunogenicity of tetanus vaccine in vitro. Sixth International Conference on Tetanus, Dec. 3-5, 1981, Lyon, Fondation Marcel Mérieux
12. UytdeHaag, F.G.C.M. et al.: Induction of antigen-specific antibody response in human peripheral blood lymphocytes in vitro by a dog kidney cell vaccine against rabies virus (DKCV). The Journal of Immunology, (1983), 131, 3, 1234-1239
13. Loggen, H.G.: Personal communication
14. UytdeHaag, F.G.C.M. et al.: Human peripheral blood lymphocytes from recently vaccinated individuals produce both type-specific and intertype cross reacting neutralizing antibody on in vitro stimulation with one type of poliovirus. The Journal of Immunology (1985), 135, 5, 3094-3101

CHAPTER 14: FINAL COMMENTS AND RECOMMENDATIONS

Most infectious diseases no longer pose major problems to human
and animal health in the Western countries. This achievement can
be largely attributed to mass active immunization. There are now
many vaccines available for both human and veterinary
application.
There exists a traditional and close relationship between the
production and quality control of these vaccines on the one hand,
and laboratory animal use on the other. In 1986, about 250,000
experimental animals were used in the Netherlands for testing
biological products, including many vaccines.
However, there are various motives which make people look for
methods which could replace, reduce and/or refine the use of
experimental animals. These so-called alternative methods are not
only desirable on ethical grounds but they are in many cases also
particularly attractive in scientific and/or economic terms.
Until recently these two latter aspects provided the chief
stimulus in the search for alternatives to animal
experimentation, and there has certainly been a considerable
reduction in the use of animals in vaccine production. However,
the ethical aspect should now be given more weight in the further
development of alternatives.
The foregoing chapters are the result of a practical approach to
the complex issue of performing experiments on live animals, and
the study was undertaken at the National Institute of Public
Health and Environmental Protection in the Netherlands.
An attempt has been made to reconcile the scientific need for
animal experimentation for the production and quality control of
vaccines with the ethical motives for replacement, reduction
and/or refinement. To this end, a survey and evaluation of the
existing guidelines for vaccine production and control have been
made, as also of the methodologies used. It can be concluded that
the potential for developing and applying methods which can
reduce and/or refine animal usage is very high. Several possible
alternatives have already been or can be applied in the
foreseeable future, while others still need more study and
validation, or discussion in a broader context. These potential
alternatives have been described in detail in chapters 8-12 of
this report. The following categories of activities are required
to achieve an effective replacement, reduction and refinement of
laboratory animal use:
A. Adaptation of the national and international guidelines;
B. Adaptation of the production techniques and planning
   schedules;
C. Validation studies;
D. Innovative research.
These categories are specified in the following summary with
reference to the chapter and section of this report in which they
have been discussed. For categories "Validation studies" and
"Innovative research" an asterisk denotes the possibilities which
- in the author's opinion - should be given priority on the basis
of their feasibility and anticipated results. This does not, of
course, imply that the other possibilities mentioned are less
important.

| A. ADAPTATION OF THE NATIONAL AND INTERNATIONAL GUIDELINES | -CHAPTER-SECTION | |

A.1.	Discontinuation of the following animal-based tests:		
A.1.a.	Test for extraneous viruses in adult and newborn mice (inactivated polio vaccine)	9	7A.3.2.
A.1.b.	Test for extraneous viruses in adult and newborn mice (live, oral polio vaccine)	9	7B.1
A.1.c.	Test for extraneous viruses in adult and newborn mice (inactivated rabies vaccine)	9	8.3.2.
A.1.d.	Test for contamination of virus suspensions with rabies virus (live vaccines for dogs and cats)	11	3.3.
A.2.	Replacement of the following animal models by either _in vitro_ or combined _in vivo_/_in vitro_ models:		
A.2.a.	Lethal challenge in guinea pigs by serum neutralization in tissue culture (diphtheria vaccine)	8	4.3.1.
A.2.b.	_In vivo_ identity test by _in vitro_ models (human bacterial vaccines) e.g.	8	3.1.
A.2.c.	Test for presence of virulent polio virus in monkeys by a test in tissue culture (US requirements for inactivated polio vaccine)	9	7A.2.
A.2.d.	Test for presence of rabies virus in mice by a test in tissue culture (inactivated rabies vaccine)	9	8.2.
A.3.	Reduction in the frequency of animal tests per vaccine batch for:		
A.3.a.	The test for specific toxicity on diphtheria vaccine	8	4.2.
A.3.b.	The test for specific toxicity on tetanus vaccine	8	6.2.
A.4.	Reduction in the number of animals for:		
A.4.a.	The test for freedom from abnormal toxicity (all human vaccines)	8	2.3.
A.4.b.	The potency test on tetanus vaccine	8	6.4.
A.4.c.	The potency test on diphtheria vaccine	8	4.3.
A.4.d.	The neurovirulence test on polio vaccine (live, oral)	9	7B.2.
A.4.e.	The test for specific toxicity on diphtheria vaccine	8	4.2.
A.4.f.	The test for specific toxicity on tetanus vaccine	8	6.2.
A.4.g.	The test for specific toxicity on cholera vaccine	8	3.2.
A.5.	Refinement of experimental techniques by:		
A.5.a.	Reduction in the frequency of taking blood samples in the testing of live poultry vaccines for extraneous microorganisms	10	2.1.1.
A.5.b.	Reduction or suppression of pain	12	10
A.5.c.	Assessment of the degree of distress both at the start and at the end of the experiment	5	4

A. ADAPTATION OF THE NATIONAL AND INTERNATIONAL   -CHAPTER-SECTION
   GUIDELINES

A.6.   Harmonization of the national and
        international guidelines and the
        establishment of a Community arbitration
        committee   12   2

A.7.   Recognition in one country of test results
        obtained in another   12   2

A.8.   Relaxation of the weight requirements for
        the animals to be used   12   7

B. ADAPTATION OF THE PRODUCTION TECHNIQUES AND   -CHAPTER-SECTION
   PLANNING SCHEDULES

B.1.   Increasing the capacity of packaging
        equipment/the volume of batches

B.2.   Combining various animal tests:
B.2.a. The safety test with the test for
        extraneous microorganisms (live poultry
        vaccines)   10   2.2.
B.2.b. The potency tests of different vaccine
        products (inactivated poultry vaccines and
        veterinary vaccines for mammals)   10   3.1/11.2
B.2.c. The potency tests of different vaccines in
        guinea pigs (inactivated vaccines for dogs,
        except the inactivated rabies vaccine)   11   3.1.2.

B.3.   Adaptation of the production techniques by:
B.3.a. Replacement of the tertiary monkey kidney
        cell cultures used for culturing and testing
        inactivated polio vaccine by Vero cells   9   7A.2.
B.3.b. Replacement of the primary rabbit kidney
        cell cultures used for culturing rubella
        vaccine by diploid cells   9   9.1.

C. VALIDATION STUDIES   -CHAPTER-SECTION

C.1.   Validation of in vitro methods to replace
        the following animal-based tests:
C.1.a. The test for absence of virulent
        mycobacteria in guinea pigs (BCG vaccine)   8   2.1.
C.1.b. The test for specific toxicity in guinea
        pigs (diphtheria vaccine)   8   4.2.
C.1.c.* The tumourigenicity test in mice and rabbits
        (human viral vaccines)   9   7.A.4.
C.1.d.* The potency test in mice (inactivated rabies
        vaccine)   9   8.4.
C.1.e.* The test for the presence of avian
        encephalomyelitis virus in chicks (live
        poultry vaccines)   10   2.1.2.

The realization of the above possibilities for replacement,
reduction and/or refinement of animal usage - the 3Rs concept -is
heavily dependent on several conditions which apply not only to
vaccine control but also to other kinds of biomedical research.

I.   Understandably, the realization of the 3Rs concept requires
      first of all more financial support. There are several good

reasons for making such an appeal, particularly to public funds. One is that the government, by establishing regulations or requirements applicable to a particular product, is responsible for most of the animal tests performed in the quality control of vaccines. Another is that there are real opportunities for reducing the use of experimental animals - so much desired by the general public - which would not receive attention without a contribution from the government. Examples include the development of in vitro methods for potency testing based on stimulation of an antibody response by antigens (e.g. the lymphocyte stimulation model discussed in chapter 8, section 4.3.3.) and the development and validation of in vitro models for the tests for specific toxicity or the presence of extraneous microorganisms. A striking feature is that financial support for the development of alternative methods in vaccine control is lagging behind that for the other areas of biomedical research in spite of their greater potential here. This can be deduced from the following survey of public grants for alternative research in the Netherlands in 1985 and 1986 (1). In addition to money from public funds, industry should also make a a substantial contribution towards the development of in vitro techniques for these will lower the costs of vaccine production and control and thus benefit industry directly.

FIELD OF SCIENTIFIC WORK	SUBSIDY, IN 1985	POUND STERLING 1986
Biotechnical research	76.000	44.000
Toxicological research	103.000	212.000
Pathological research	97.000	25.000
Immunological research (incl. vaccines)	42.000	42.000

II. There are various scientific organizations whose main objective is to promote the concept of the 3 Rs -Replacement, Reduction and Refinement. They stimulate and coordinate alternatives research by raising and distributing public money, and promote the application of new in vitro techniques. Examples of such organizations are: the Johns Hopkins Center in the USA, FRAME (Fund for the Replacement of Animals in Medical Experiments) in the UK, and ERGATT (European Research Group for Alternatives to Toxicity Testing) in Europe. Nearly all these organizations are concerned only with toxicity testing. There is not one organization dealing specifically with biological products, despite the advances being made in this field. It would therefore seem desirable to create an organization for promoting and coordinating research into alternatives to animal experiments on an international level, possibly in cooperation with the FDA, WHO and/or the European Pharmacopoeia authorities. This could be instigated by a group of scientists engaged in vaccine production and control and interested in the 3 Rs concept. Such an organization could also promote the international validation studies. A newly developed alternative method is all too frequently not incorporated into the international and

supranational regulations because of lack of financial
resources, capacity and/or organization for initiating and
coordinating validation studies.

III. Animal experimentation can become a practice taken for
granted, especially when it is of a routine nature and/or
regulated by law, so that often no consideration is given to
the suffering inflicted on the animals concerned. It is
therefore advisable - not least on economic grounds - to re-
evaluate periodically the possibilities for reduction and/or
refinement of the existing animal tests. To date, the
institutes have lacked the time and resources to do justice
to these aspects. Special facilities, created for this by
the government, could as a first task evaluate periodically
that part of the quality control covered by the regulations,
such as toxicity testing, vaccine control, testing of other
biological products (e.g. biotechnology-derived products)
and pharmacological research and testing.
The effective re-evaluation of existing animal tests also
requires a certain flexibility on the part of the control
authorities in the adaptation of the national and
international guidelines. It is the government's obligation
to exert its influence in this respect and to prevent
innovative research from becoming buried under red tape.

IV. Partly related to the last point is the recommendation to
establish a central database on alternatives research and
alternative techniques. Advances in the field of reduction
and refinement of animal use are being made in all branches
of biomedical research and are usually published in
specialist journals. This can obstruct the effective
exchange of data and information, which could be overcome by
setting up a data bank. Such a databank could contribute to
a more efficient transfer of knowledge from fundamental
scientific research to applied research. It could also fill
a social need by providing objective information about the
possibilit ies and impossibilities of alternative methods.

V. The basic reason for the intensive quality control of
vaccines is society's demand for safe and reliable products.
This social pressure is very strong in comparison with other
risks being taken in everyday life and has contributed to
the current extensive use of experimental animals. Yet, this
fact is all too frequently overlooked in discussions about
the background of animal experimentation. As a result, there
is a tendency to place all the responsibility for reducing
the use of experimental animals on those who are directly
involved in animal experimentation. If a further reduction
in laboratory animal use is to be achieved, it will be
useful to take both the public concern for animal welfare
and the demand for absolutely safe products into
consideration.

EPILOGUE

Although scientific organizations, industry, the government and
animal societies do not share a unified position on animal
experimentation, there is one concern about which they all agree,
namely, the desire for a well-founded replacement, reduction or
refinement of laboratory animal use. The fact that this desire

may be motivated by different interests is not relevant here. Reducing animal usage is a complex matter for which there are generally no easy and ready-made solutions. Yet, the advantages to be expected from such a reduction are in many respects great enough to merit intensification of research in this direction. It requires the efforts of many people from all sectors of society. In the belief that consultations, based on what unites the government, scientific community, industry and animal protection societies, will ultimately give better results than those based on what separates them, a plea is made for constructive cooperation. This requires not only an unprejudiced attitude but also adequate information transfer. It is hoped that this report may have contributed towards this goal.

REFERENCE

1. Animal Experimentation Policy, Lower House, 1985-86 Session, Document 18,450, No. 10, the Netherlands

158

This report would not have been possible without the financial
support of five Dutch animal protection societies, namely:
- de Anti-Vivisectie Stichting (AVS);
- de Nederlandse Bond tot Bestrijding van de Vivisectie (NBBV);
- de Nederlandse Vereniging tot Bescherming van Dieren;
- de Stichting Bevordering Alternatieven voor Dierproeven (BAVD);
- de Stichting Schoonheid zonder Wreedheid (SSZW);
and from the Ministry of Welfare, Public Health and Culture.